Seizures

Guest Editors

ANDY JAGODA, MD
EDWARD P. SLOAN, MD, MPH

EMERGENCY MEDICINE CLINICS OF NORTH AMERICA

www.emed.theclinics.com

Consulting Editor
AMAL MATTU, MD

February 2011 • Volume 29 • Number 1

SAUNDERS an imprint of ELSEVIER, Inc.

W.B. SAUNDERS COMPANY

A Division of Elsevier Inc.

1600 John F. Kennedy Boulevard ● Suite 1800 ● Philadelphia, Pennsylvania 19103-2899

http://www.theclinics.com

EMERGENCY MEDICINE CLINICS OF NORTH AMERICA Volume 29, Number 1
February 2011 ISSN 0733-8627, ISBN-13: 978-1-4557-0438-5

Editor: Patrick Manley
Developmental Editor: Donald Mumford

Photocopying
Single photocopies of single articles may be made for personal use as allowed by national copyright laws. Permission of the Publisher and payment of a fee is required for all other photocopying, including multiple or systematic copying, copying for advertising or promotional purposes, resale, and all forms of document delivery. Special rates are available for educational institutions that wish to make photocopies for non-profit educational classroom use. For information on how to seek permission visit www.elsevier.com/permissions or call: (+44) 1865 843830 (UK)/(+1) 215 239 3804 (USA).

Derivative Works
Subscribers may reproduce tables of contents or prepare lists of articles including abstracts for internal circulation within their institutions. Permission of the Publisher is required for resale or distribution outside the institution. Permission of the Publisher is required for all other derivative works, including compilations and translations (please consult www.elsevier.com/permissions).

Electronic Storage or Usage
Permission of the Publisher is required to store or use electronically any material contained in this journal, including any article or part of an article (please consult www.elsevier.com/permissions). Except as outlined above, no part of this publication may be reproduced, stored in a retrieval system or transmitted in any form or by any means, electronic, mechanical, photocopying, recording or otherwise, without prior written permission of the Publisher.

Notice
No responsibility is assumed by the Publisher for any injury and/or damage to persons or property as a matter of products liability, negligence or otherwise, or from any use or operation of any methods, products, instructions or ideas contained in the material herein. Because of rapid advances in the medical sciences, in particular, independent verification of diagnoses and drug dosages should be made.

Although all advertising material is expected to conform to ethical (medical) standards, inclusion in this publication does not constitute a guarantee or endorsement of the quality or value of such product or of the claims made of it by its manufacturer.

Emergency Medicine Clinics of North America (ISSN 0733-8627) is published quarterly by Elsevier Inc., 360 Park Avenue South, New York, NY, 10010-1710. Months of issue are February, May, August, and November. Business and Editorial Offices: 1600 John F. Kennedy Boulevard, Suite 1800, Philadelphia, PA 19103-2899. Customer Service Office: 6277 Sea Harbor Drive, Orlando, FL 32887-4800. Periodicals postage paid at New York, NY, and additional mailing offices. Subscription prices are $133.00 per year (US students), $264.00 per year (US individuals), $455.00 per year (US institutions), $189.00 per year (international students), $379.00 per year (international individuals), $549.00 per year (international institutions), $189.00 per year (Canadian students), $326.00 per year (Canadian individuals), and $549.00 per year (Canadian institutions). International air speed delivery is included in all *Clinics'* subscription prices. All prices are subject to change without notice. **POSTMASTER:** Send address changes to *Emergency Medicine Clinics of North America*, Elsevier Periodicals Customer Service, 11830 Westline Industrial Drive, St. Louis, MO 63146. Customer Service (orders, claims, online, change of address): Elsevier Periodicals Customer Service, 11830 Westline Industrial Drive, St. Louis, MO 63146. Tel: 1-800-654-2452 (U.S. and Canada); 314-453-7041 (outside U.S. and Canada). Fax: 314-453-5170. E-mail: journalscustomerservice-usa@elsevier.com (for print support); journalsonlinesupport-usa@elsevier.com (for online support).

Reprints. For copies of 100 or more of articles in this publication, please contact the Commercial Reprints Department, Elsevier Inc., 360 Park Avenue South, New York, NY 10010-1710. Tel.: 212-633-3812; Fax: 212-462-1935; E-mail: reprints@elsevier.com.

Emergency Medicine Clinics of North America is covered in *MEDLINE/PubMed (Index Medicus), Current Contents/Clinical Medicine, EMBASE/Excerpta Medica, BIOSIS, SciSearch, CINAHL, ISI/BIOMED,* and *Research Alert.*

Printed and bound by CPI Group (UK) Ltd, Croydon, CR0 4YY

Transferred to Digital Print 2011

Contributors

CONSULTING EDITOR

AMAL MATTU, MD, FAAEM, FACEP
Program Director, Emergency Medicine Residency; Professor, Department of Emergency Medicine, University of Maryland School of Medicine, Baltimore, Maryland

GUEST EDITORS

ANDY JAGODA, MD, FACEP
Professor and Chair, Department Emergency Medicine, Mount Sinai Hospital, Mount Sinai School of Medicine, New York, New York

EDWARD P. SLOAN, MD, MPH, FACEP
Professor and Director of Research, Department of Emergency Medicine, University of Illinois at Chicago School of Medicine; President, Foundation for Education and Research in Neurologic Emergencies, Chicago, Illinois

AUTHORS

ANDREW K. CHANG, MD, MS
Associate Professor, Department of Emergency Medicine, Albert Einstein College of Medicine; Attending Physician, Montefiore Medical Center, Bronx, New York

NATHAN B. FOUNTAIN, MD
Professor of Neurology; Director, Comprehensive Epilepsy Program, Department of Neurology, University of Virginia Health System, Charlottesville, Virginia

JOSHUA N. GOLDSTEIN, MD, PhD
Harvard-Affiliated Emergency Medicine Residency; Department of Emergency Medicine, Massachusetts General Hospital; Harvard Medical School, Boston, Massachusetts

KANIKA GUPTA, MD
Department of Emergency Medicine, Mount Sinai Hospital, Mount Sinai School of Medicine, New York, New York

LOUIS C. HAMPERS, MD, MBA
Assistant Professor of Pediatrics, Section of Pediatric Emergency Medicine, University of Colorado School of Medicine; Medical Director, Emergency Department, The Children's Hospital, Denver, Colorado

PHYLLIS L. HENDRY, MD, FAAP, FACEP
Assistant Chair, Emergency Medicine Research, Department of Emergency Medicine; Associate Professor of Emergency Medicine and Pediatrics, University of Florida College of Medicine, Jacksonville, Florida

ROBERT J. HOFFMAN, MD
Research Director, Department of Emergency Medicine, Beth Israel Medical Center,
New York, New York

J. STEPHEN HUFF, MD
Associate Professor of Emergency Medicine and Neurology, Department of Emergency
Medicine, University of Virginia Health System, Charlottesville, Virginia

OLIVER L. HUNG, MD
Department of Emergency Medicine, Morristown Memorial Hospital, Morristown,
New Jersey

ANDY JAGODA, MD, FACEP
Professor and Chair, Department of Emergency Medicine, Mount Sinai Hospital,
Mount Sinai School of Medicine, New York, New York

JONATHAN L. LISS, MD
Diplomat, American Academy of Neurology, Department of Emergency Services,
The Medical Center, Columbus, Georgia

JENNIFER L. MARTINDALE, MD
Department of Emergency Medicine, Brigham and Women's Hospital; Division
of Emergency Medicine, Children's Hospital; Harvard-Affiliated Emergency Medicine
Residency; Department of Emergency Medicine, Massachusetts General Hospital;
Harvard Medical School, Boston, Massachusetts

DAVID MCMICKEN, MD, FACEP
Department of Emergency Services, The Medical Center, Columbus, Georgia

ROLAND C. MERCHANT, MD, MPH, ScD
Associate Professor, Departments of Emergency Medicine and Community Health,
Rhode Island Hospital, Alpert Medical School of Brown University, Providence,
Rhode Island

GLEN E. MICHAEL, MD
Clinical Instructor, Department of Emergency Medicine, University of Virginia School
of Medicine, Charlottesville, Virginia

ROBERT E. O'CONNOR, MD, MPH
Professor and Chair, Department of Emergency Medicine, University of Virginia School
of Medicine, Charlottesville, Virginia

DANIEL J. PALLIN, MD, MPH
Department of Emergency Medicine, Brigham and Women's Hospital; Division
of Emergency Medicine, Children's Hospital; Harvard-Affiliated Emergency Medicine
Residency; Harvard Medical School, Boston, Massachusetts

JAMES RIVIELLO, MD
Department of Emergency Medicine, Mount Sinai School of Medicine, New York,
New York; Department of Emergency Medicine, University of Illinois College of Medicine,
Chicago, Illinois

GHAZALA Q. SHARIEFF, MD, FACEP, FAAEM
Department of Emergency Medicine, Palomar-Pomerado Health System/California
Emergency Physicians; Professor of Pediatrics, University of California,
San Diego, California

ADHI N. SHARMA, MD
Chairman, Department of Emergency Medicine, Good Samaritan Hospital Medical Center, West Islip; Assistant Professor, Department of Emergency Medicine, Mount Sinai School of Medicine, New York, New York

PETER SHEARER, MD
Assistant Professor, Department of Emergency Medicine, Mount Sinai School of Medicine, New York, New York; Department of Emergency Medicine, University of Illinois College of Medicine, Chicago, Illinois

RICHARD D. SHIH, MD
Department of Emergency Medicine, Morristown Memorial Hospital, Morristown, New Jersey

SHLOMO SHINNAR, MD, PhD
Professor of Neurology, Pediatrics and Epidemiology and Population Health; Hyman Climenko Professor of Neuroscience Research; Director, Comprehensive Epilepsy Management Center, Montefiore Medical Center, Albert Einstein College of Medicine, Bronx, New York

MATTHEW S. SIKET, MD, MS
Department of Emergency Medicine, Rhode Island Hospital, Alpert Medical School of Brown University, Providence, Rhode Island

LOUIS A. SPINA, MD
Fellowship Director Pediatric Emergency Medicine; Assistant Professor of Emergency Medicine and Pediatrics, Division of Pediatric Emergency Medicine, Department of Emergency Medicine, Mount Sinai Medical Center, New York, New York

LATHA GANTI STEAD, MD, MS, FACEP
Professor and Chief, Division of Clinical Research, Department of Emergency Medicine, University of Florida College of Medicine, Gainesville, Florida; Adjunct Professor, Department of Emergency Medicine, Mayo Clinic College of Medicine, Rochester, Minnesota

Contents

J. Stephen Huff and Nathan B. Fountain

The pathophysiology of seizures is multifactorial and incompletely understood. Experimental work demonstrates that prolonged, abnormal, and
excessive neuronal electrical activity in itself is injurious through several
mechanisms independent of systemic acidosis and hypoxia. Population
survival studies and laboratory investigations support the idea that brain
injury and epileptogenesis result from status epilepticus. The basic distinction in seizure types is that of generalized and partial seizures. Correct
classification of seizure types will aid in clinical communications and guide
correct therapies. Revised definitions of generalized convulsive status epilepticus suggest making this diagnosis with as few as 5 minutes of continuous seizure activity.

Jennifer L. Martindale, Joshua N. Goldstein, and Daniel J. Pallin

Although only 3% of people in the United States are diagnosed with
epilepsy, 11% will have at least one seizure during their lifetime. Seizures
account for about 1% of all emergency department (ED) visits, and about
2% of visits to children's hospital EDs. Seizure accounts for about 3% of
prehospital transports. In adult ED patients, common causes of seizure are
alcoholism, stroke, tumor, trauma, and central nervous system infection. In
children, febrile seizures are most common. In infants younger than
6 months, hyponatremia and infection are important considerations.
Epilepsy is an uncommon cause of seizures in the ED, accounting for
a minority of seizure-related visits. Of ED patients with seizure, about
7% have status epilepticus, which has an age-dependent mortality aver-
aging 22%.

Glen E. Michael and Robert E. O'Connor

Seizure is one of the most common complaints encountered in the prehospital setting. In this review the authors discuss the prehospital management of seizures and review the evidence for specific treatment
approaches. Specific attention is devoted to prehospital care of the pediatric seizure patient. Topics of interest to Emergency Medical Services
directors such as patient refusal, resource allocation, and dispatch priority
are also addressed.

Up to 5% of the population will experience at least 1 nonfebrile seizure at some point during their lifetime. The management of a patient who has had a first-time seizure is driven by the history and physical examination. In almost one-half of these patients, the cause of their seizure is not identified. In general, patients with comorbidities, a focal neurologic examination, or who have not returned to a normal baseline mental status require an extensive diagnostic evaluation including a noncontrast head computed tomography (CT) scan in the emergency department (ED). Adults with a first-time seizure, with no comorbidities, and who have returned to a normal baseline require only serum glucose and electrolyte determination. Women of reproductive age also require a pregnancy test. Patients with a normal neurologic examination, normal laboratory results, and no signs of structural brain disease do not require hospitalization or antiepileptic medications. Initiation of antiepileptic therapy depends on the assessed risk for recurrence, in conjunction with a neurologist consultation.

Generalized convulsive status epilepticus (GCSE) has a high morbidity and mortality, such that the rapid delivery of anticonvulsant therapy should be initiated within minutes of seizure onset to prevent permanent neuronal damage. GCSE is not a specific disease but is a manifestation of either a primary central nervous system (CNS) insult or a systemic disorder with secondary CNS effects. It is mandatory to look for an underlying cause. First-line therapies for seizures and status epilepticus include the use of a benzodiazepine, followed by an infusion of a phenytoin with a possible role for intravenous valproate or phenobarbital. If these first-line medications fail to terminate the GCSE, treatment includes the continuous infusion of midazolam, pentobarbital, or propofol.

Nonconvulsive status epilepticus (NCSE) refers to a prolonged seizure that manifests primarily as altered mental status as opposed to the dramatic convulsions seen in generalized tonic-clonic status epilepticus. There are 2 main types of NCSE, each of which has a different presentation, cause, and expected outcome. In the first type of NCSE, patients present with confusion or abnormal behavior, suggesting the diagnosis of absence status epilepticus (ASE) or complex partial status epilepticus (CPSE). The second type of NCSE (subtle status epilepticus [SSE]) must be considered in comatose patients who present after a prolonged generalized tonic-clonic seizure and who may have only subtle motor manifestations of a seizure, such as facial or hand twitchings. Whereas the morbidity and mortality in patients with prolonged ASE or CPSE is low, the mortality associated with SSE can exceed 30% if the seizure duration is greater than 60 minutes.

Patients with psychogenic (nonepileptic) seizures (PS) are frequently encountered by clinicians in the emergency medicine setting. Despite the tendency for these patients to seek frequent medical attention, the time between onset of symptoms and diagnosis is often more than 7 years. The cause of PS is multifactorial, but most patients are thought to have an underlying dissociative condition. The diagnostic evaluation in the emergency department is challenging and relies heavily on clinical suspicion, based on historical and physical features. Laboratory testing and therapeutic maneuvers are of limited utility; prolonged video electroencephalography is the diagnostic gold standard. Once the diagnosis has been secured, the mainstay of treatment involves addressing the underlying psychological distress.

Febrile seizures are common in children, who are often brought to the nearest emergency department (ED). Patients who meet the case definition of simple febrile seizure are not at higher risk for serious bacterial illness than clinically similar febrile children who have not experienced a convulsion. Children who have had complex febrile seizures must be evaluated on a case-by-case basis, and treated with diagnostic and therapeutic measures based on the differential diagnosis. Round-the-clock prophylactic administration of antipyretics has not been demonstrated to affect recurrence of simple febrile seizure. Parents should be informed that recurrence is common, and that these convulsions are benign with an excellent prognosis. Care-givers should be informed that the risk of developing epilepsy after a simple febrile seizure is low, but that complex febrile seizures carry a significantly higher risk.

Most well-appearing children who have had an afebrile seizure can be managed as outpatients with instructions for an outpatient electroencephalogram and primary care physician follow-up. Laboratory studies are needed only in children younger than 6 months, in patients with prolonged seizures or altered level of consciousness, or in those with history of a metabolic disorder or dehydration. Emergent neuroimaging is not recommended in children with a first unprovoked afebrile seizure, although studies should be considered in children with a predisposing condition or focal seizures if younger than 3 years.

The physical and emotional stress of pregnancy can precipitate new-onset seizures in a woman. In these cases, emergency department evaluations must rule out underlying pathology. Careful consideration of antiepileptic drug use must be considered in the first trimester as all antiepileptic drugs have been linked to some teratogenic effect. Eclampsia must always be considered in the pregnant woman who is more than 20 weeks gestation; 25% of eclamptic seizures occur in the postpartum period. Magnesium is the recommended treatment for eclamptic seizures when delivery is not possible.

The term alcohol-related seizures (ARS) is used to refer to all seizures in the aggregate associated with alcohol use, including the subset of alcohol withdrawal seizures (AWS). From 20% to 40% of patients with seizure who present to an emergency department have seizures related to alcohol abuse. However, it is critical to avoid prematurely labeling a seizure as being caused by alcohol withdrawal before performing a careful diagnostic evaluation. Benzodiazepines alone are sufficient to prevent AWS. The alcoholic patient with a documented history of ARS, who experiences a single seizure or a short burst of seizures should be treated with lorazepam, 2 mg intravenously.

Toxin-related seizures result from an imbalance in the brain's equilibrium of excitation-inhibition. Fortunately, most toxin-related seizures respond to standard therapy using benzodiazepines. However, a few alterations in the standard approach are recommended to ensure optimal care and expedient termination of seizure activity. If 2 doses of a benzodiazepine do not terminate the seizure activity, a therapeutic dose of pyridoxine (5 g intravenously in an adult and 70 mg/kg intravenously in a child) should be considered. Phenytoin should be avoided because it is ineffective for many toxin-induced seizures and is potentially harmful when used to treat seizures induced by theophylline or cyclic antidepressants.

During the past decade several new antiepileptic drugs (AEDs) have become available, including new formulations of some of the older medications. Understanding the pharmacokinetics of the new AEDs is important because they are primarily used for adjunctive therapy and interactions with other medications can result in significant toxicities. The new-generation AEDs do not cause serious morbidity in overdose, and treatment is primarily supportive. Specific medications should be chosen based on the patient's history and presentation.

THE CLINICS ARE NOW AVAILABLE ONLINE!

Access your subscription at:
www.theclinics.com

GOAL STATEMENT

The goal of *Emergency Medicine Clinics of North America* is to keep practicing physicians up to date with current clinical practice in emergency medicine by providing timely articles reviewing the state of the art in patient care.

ACCREDITATION

The *Emergency Medical Clinics of North America* is planned and implemented in accordance with the Essential Areas and Policies of the Accreditation Council for Continuing Medical Education (ACCME) through the joint sponsorship of the University of Virginia School of Medicine and Elsevier. The University of Virginia School of Medicine is accredited by the ACCME to provide continuing medical education for physicians.

The University of Virginia School of Medicine designates this educational activity for a maximum of 15 *AMA PRA Category 1 Credits*™ for each issue, 60 credits per year. Physicians should only claim credit commensurate with the extent of their participation in the activity.

The American Medical Association has determined that physicians not licensed in the US who participate in this CME activity are eligible for a maximum of 15 *AMA PRA Category 1 Credits*™ for each issue, 60 credits per year.

The Emergency Medicine Clinics of North America CME program is approved by the American College of Emergency Physicians for 60 hours of ACEP Category I Credit per year.

Credit can be earned by reading the text material, taking the CME examination online at http://www.theclinics.com/home/cme, and completing the evaluation. After taking the test, you will be required to review any and all incorrect answers. Following completion of the test and evaluation, your credit will be awarded and you may print your certificate.

FACULTY DISCLOSURE/CONFLICT OF INTEREST

The University of Virginia School of Medicine, as an ACCME accredited provider, endorses and strives to comply with the Accreditation Council for Continuing Medical Education (ACCME) Standards of Commercial Support, Commonwealth of Virginia statutes, University of Virginia policies and procedures, and associated federal and private regulations and guidelines on the need for disclosure and monitoring of proprietary and financial interests that may affect the scientific integrity and balance of content delivered in continuing medical education activities under our auspices.

The University of Virginia School of Medicine requires that all CME activities accredited through this institution be developed independently and be scientifically rigorous, balanced and objective in the presentation/discussion of its content, theories and practices.

All authors/editors participating in an accredited CME activity are expected to disclose to the readers relevant financial relationships with commercial entities occurring within the past 12 months (such as grants or research support, employee, consultant, stock holder, member of speakers bureau, etc.). The University of Virginia School of Medicine will employ appropriate mechanisms to resolve potential conflicts of interest to maintain the standards of fair and balanced education to the reader. Questions about specific strategies can be directed to the Office of Continuing Medical Education, University of Virginia School of Medicine, Charlottesville, Virginia.

The faculty and staff of the University of Virginia Office of Continuing Medical Education have no financial affiliations to disclose.

The authors/editors listed below have identified no professional or financial affiliations for themselves or their spouse/partner:

Andrew K. Chang, MD, MS; Louis C. Hampers, MD, MBA; Robert J. Hoffman, MD; J. Stephen Huff, MD; Oliver L. Hung, MD; Andy Jagoda, MD (Guest Editor); Patrick Manley, (Acquisitions Editor); Jennifer L. Martindale, MD; Amal Mattu, MD (Consulting Editor); David McMicken, MD; Roland C. Merchant, MD, MPH, ScD; Glen E. Michael, MD; Robert E. O'Connor, MD, MPH; Daniel J. Pallin, MD, MPH; Adhi N. Sharma, MD; Peter Shearer, MD; Richard D. Shih, MD; Matthew S. Siket, MD, MS; Edward P. Sloan, MD, MPH (Guest Editor); Louis A. Spina, MD; Latha Ganti Stead, MD, MS; and Bill Woods, MD (Test Author).

The authors/editors listed below have identified the following professional or financial affiliations for themselves of their spouse/partner:

Nathan B. Fountain, MD is an industry funded research/investigator for UCB, Vertex, Neurpace, and Medtronic.
Joshua N. Goldstein, MD, PhD is a consultant and is on the Advisory Committee/Board for CSL Behring.
Kanika Gupta, MD is employed by Mount Sinai.
Jonathan L. Liss, MD is an industry funded research/investigator and consultant, and is on the Speakers' Bureau and Advisory Committee/Board, for Pfizer, BI, Lilly, Jensan, GSK, Sepracor, and Forrest.
James Riviello, MD's spouse is Section Editor for Up To Date.
Shlomo Shinnar, MD, PhD is on the Speakers' Bureau for UCB Pharma.

Disclosure of Discussion of Non-FDA Approved Uses for Pharmaceutical Products and/or Medical Devices.
The University of Virginia School of Medicine, as an ACCME provider, requires that all faculty presenters identify and disclose any off-label uses for pharmaceutical and medical device products. The University of Virginia School of Medicine recommends that each physician fully review all the available data on new products or procedures prior to clinical use.

TO ENROLL

To enroll in the Emergency Medicine Clinics of North America Continuing Medical Education program, call customer service at 1-800-654-2452 or visit us online at www.theclinics.com/home/cme. The CME program is available to subscribers for an additional fee of $190.00.

Foreword

Seizures

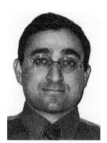

Amal Mattu, MD
Consulting Editor

Seizures have been a source of mystery and intrigue to medical and laypeople alike for thousands of years. The first book on epilepsy, *On the Sacred Disease*, was written by Hippocrates in 400 BC, and since that time, medical writers and physicians have attempted to identify, understand, and treat the condition. Many famous historical figures have been suspected of having seizures, including Socrates, Julius Caesar, Napoleon, and Lenin. Many modern-day celebrities have suffered from seizures and epilepsy as well, such as Budd Abbott, Danny Glover, Lindsey Buckingham, Prince, and Florence Griffith Joyner, among many, many others. Seizures are a condition that almost every adult member of our society has heard of and would identify if they witnessed one ... such is the prevalence and prominence of the condition in our society. Yet, despite the prevalence and "drama" of the condition, we still lack a full understanding of the condition, and we also lack ideal therapies to prevent and treat the condition. The mainstay of therapy since the 1940s has been phenytoin, but side effects have somewhat limited its utility. Other therapies have been criticized as being too sedating or too slow-acting. More than 2000 years after its first medical description, seizures remain a common condition with imperfect therapies and a still uncertain etiology in many patients. However, some recent advances in our understanding of pathophysiology as well as recent advances in pharmacological management have provided great promise for the future management of this condition.

In this issue of *Emergency Medicine Clinics of North America*, Guest Editors Drs Ed Sloane and Andy Jagoda, two leading educators in the area of neurologic emergencies, have assembled an outstanding team to teach us about the latest advances in emergency diagnosis and management of seizures. The authors address basic background information such as epidemiology as well as new understandings regarding the pathophysiology underlying seizures. Articles are devoted to helping us properly define and classify the various types of seizures. Seizures in "special groups" such as pregnant patients and pediatric patients are addressed, and non-epilepsy-related seizures such as psychogenic, alcohol-related, and toxin-related seizures are addressed as

Emerg Med Clin N Am 29 (2011) xiii–xiv
doi:10.1016/j.emc.2010.10.003

well. Articles are specifically devoted to pediatric seizures, including febrile and afebrile seizures. An informative article discusses old and new drugs for management of these patients. Most important to emergency physicians are additional articles devoted to treatment of convulsive and nonconvulsive status epilepticus.

The Guest Editors and authors are to be commended for their hard work. This issue of *Clinics* is the most comprehensive text that I've ever encountered devoted to the emergent management of patients with seizures. I feel confident in stating that any provider that reads this issue will certainly be as much of an expert as any practicing neurologist in caring for patients with single, repetitive, or ongoing seizures. I strongly recommend mastery of this material, and you'd certainly be doing your colleagues in neurology a service by handing them a copy of the text as well. Kudos to the Guest Editors and their authors on their outstanding work!

Amal Mattu, MD
Department of Emergency Medicine
University of Maryland School of Medicine
110 South Paca Street, 6th Floor, Suite 200
Baltimore, MD 21201, USA

E-mail address:
amattu@smail.umaryland.edu

Preface

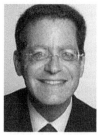 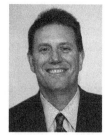

Andy Jagoda, MD   Edward P. Sloan, MD, MPH
Guest Editors

Seizures and status epilepticus (SE) are neurologic emergencies that occur frequently in the prehospital and Emergency Department (ED) settings. The majority of patients who have had an acute seizure or who are in SE are treated in the ED; thus, emergency physicians play a critical role in their resuscitation. Patients who are actively seizing require prompt diagnosis, treatment, and seizure termination in order to minimize morbidity and maximize outcomes. Acute care providers, including paramedics, nurses, and physicians, must consider the etiology of the event, provide diagnostic testing, provide anti-epileptic drugs (AEDs) and other interventions when indicated, and determine the appropriate disposition for the patient. In order to do so, the epidemiology, differential diagnosis, and likely outcome of the seizure must be taken into consideration. It is necessary to recognize the different types of seizures, including generalized convulsive status epeilepticus, nonconvulsive status epilepticus, and psychogenic seizures, and to be aware of the protocols and guidelines that define best practice. Key to seizure management is often the identification and treatment of comorbid conditions including brain injury (acute stroke and trauma), alcohol and toxins, pregnancy, and metabolic disorders. Last, seizure management is on a continuum through the health care system; thus, the prehospital provider and emergency physician must be prepared to communicate and hand off care to other providers in the system.

The Foundation for Education and Research in Neurologic Emergencies (FERNE) was created with a mission to promote the delivery of care to patients with neurologic emergencies. FERNE initially received grant funding from Parke-Davis in 1997 to develop an emergency medicine resource for prehospital and ED research and education in neurologic emergencies. Over the past thirteen years FERNE has secured additional funding from a large variety of sources that have resulted in research fellowships, conferences, educational materials, and web-based products. Over 250 emergency physicians have educated their peers through FERNE, and the FERNE website (www.ferne.org) is accessed over three million times a year.

Seizures and status epilepticus have been a focus of many of FERNE's activities and led to the interest in publishing a seizure-related primer. Initially FERNE conceived the product as a journal supplement and received support from Eisai, Inc. for the

Emerg Med Clin N Am 29 (2011) xv–xvi
doi:10.1016/j.emc.2010.10.002
0733-8627/11/$ – see front matter © 2011 Elsevier Inc. All rights reserved.

emed.theclinics.com

administrative costs related to the project. Unforeseen delays resulted in putting the project on hold; however, thanks to the willingness of the *Emergency Medicine Clinics of North America* publishing group, FERNE is pleased to be able to publish this issue on "Seizures in the Emergency Department."

This issue of *Emergency Medicine Clinics of North America* features state-of-the-art reviews on essential seizure-related topics that are encountered in the ED. The articles on epidemiology and seizure classification provide the foundation needed to understand how and why seizures occur, thus providing a pathophysiologic base to understanding diagnostic and treatment strategies. The prehospital article addresses the special circumstances that govern the care of seizure and SE patients in the out-of-hospital setting. The first-time seizure in the ED review addresses the unique questions that guide the management of patients with a first-time seizure, such as who to admit and whether or not to initiate AED therapies. The succeeding articles address a variety of emergency medicine focused topics ranging from status epileptics, to febrile seizures, to alcohol, and to pregnancy-related seizures. The final article provides an update on the new AEDs that emergency physicians may encounter both in therapeutic and in overdose settings. These reviews are intended to provide an evidence-based examination of the clinical problems related to seizures and the acute interventions that will maximize the effectiveness of neuro-resuscitation in the ED. These reviews are ultimately intended to promote quality acute patient management and to stimulate innovations and research in the care of patients with neurologic emergencies.

In conclusion, emergency physicians play a key role in the diagnosis and acute management of patients with acute seizures and SE. The resuscitation of the seizing patient requires a simultaneous, coordinated approach that includes patient stabilization, timely and efficient diagnostic testing, and effective pharmacologic intervention. It is hoped that this *Emergency Medicine Clinics of North America* volume will provide a useful resource that will enhance understanding, optimize patient resuscitation and outcomes, and improve the clinical practice in both the prehospital and the ED settings.

Andy Jagoda, MD
Department of Emergency Medicine
Mount Sinai Hospital
Mount Sinai School of Medicine
One Gustave Levy Place, Box 1620
New York, NY 10029, USA

Edward P. Sloan, MD, MPH
Department of Emergency Medicine
University of Illinois at Chicago School of Medicine
471H, CME, (MC 724)
808 South Wood Street
Chicago, IL 60612-7354, USA

E-mail addresses:
Andy.Jagoda@mountsinai.org (A. Jagoda)
edsloanuic@gmail.com (E.P. Sloan)

Pathophysiology and Definitions of Seizures and Status Epilepticus

J. Stephen Huff, MD[a],*, Nathan B. Fountain, MD[b]

KEYWORDS

- Seizures • Status epilepticus • Epileptic syndromes
- Seizure classification

Seizures represent the effects of abnormal electrical discharges of cortical neurons. Every individual has the capacity to have a seizure. The question that begs for an answer is how does a seizure first arise? Taking this to the cellular level, what mechanism or mechanisms cause a group of neurons to manifest this abnormal physiologic response? The traditional model is that large groups of hyperexcitable neurons become coordinated in their actions and recruit adjacent neurons in a synchronized flurry of discharges. Many different mechanisms are thought to be involved in this process, from a simple genetic predisposition to seizures to specific pathophysiologic mechanisms at the extracellular, cellular, and subcellular levels.

PATHOPHYSIOLOGY

Provoked seizures can occur in anyone and do not constitute epilepsy. The terms secondary seizures or acute symptomatic seizures are sometimes used to describe seizures from a variety of identifiable causes, eg, electrolyte abnormalities, toxins, and tumors. Epilepsy is present when seizures occur without a provoking factor because of an enduring tendency to seizures. Altered brain physiology is always present in patients with epilepsy, yet seizures occur essentially at random for entirely unknown reasons. Nevertheless, some basic physiologic abnormalities causing the underlying tendency for seizures to occur are known.

Seizures do not occur spontaneously under normal circumstances because neuronal physiology maintains the stability of neuronal membranes and prevents rapid

[a] Department of Emergency Medicine, University of Virginia Health System, Box 800699, Charlottesville, VA 22908, USA
[b] Comprehensive Epilepsy Program, Department of Neurology, University of Virginia Health System, Box 800394, Charlottesville, VA 22908, USA
* Corresponding author.
E-mail address: jsh5n@virginia.edu

Emerg Med Clin N Am 29 (2011) 1–13
doi:10.1016/j.emc.2010.08.001
0733-8627/11/$ – see front matter © 2011 Elsevier Inc. All rights reserved.

transfer of the synchronous discharges that initiate a seizure. Several remarkable normal mechanisms allow only a single action potential to pass in a time interval from one neuron to the next as part of normal synaptic information transfer. Seizures can be provoked in a normal brain by circumstances that disrupt this stability. For example, alterations of ion concentrations, such as hyponatremia, cause a loss of the normal electrochemical gradients across cell membranes that are needed to maintain stability; drug withdrawal from benzodiazepines, barbiturates, and especially alcohol probably cause inhibitory $GABA_A$ receptors to be sensitized so that neuronal activity that is normally harmless stimulates a seizure; hypoglycemia alters cellular metabolism.

The propensity to have a seizure can result from abnormalities affecting almost any level of the nervous system—ions, receptors, cells, networks, or whole brain regions—and may vary with seizure type or epilepsy syndrome. Generalized tonic-clonic seizures arise in patients with some types of "idiopathic generalized epilepsy" because of abnormalities of sodium channels, or more rarely calcium channels.[1] "Autosomal dominant nocturnal frontal lobe epilepsy," another epilepsy syndrome, is attributable to mutations in the acetylcholine receptor.[2] The most common form of temporal lobe epilepsy is associated with abnormalities of cellular growth in which specific cells in the temporal lobe sprout new growth that then paradoxically turn around to connect back onto themselves, leading to self-excitation.[3] Local brain malformations are the most obvious example of abnormal networks of cells causing seizures; it is thought that aberrant connections of misdirected neurons leads to seizures, but this is still unknown and the subject of intense recent research.[4]

Although the pathophysiological mechanisms of some types of epilepsy are known, similar treatments are aimed at stopping seizures or reducing the tendency for occurrence regardless of the cause. Most antiepileptic drugs (AEDs) were found fortuitously and their mechanism of action is unknown and therefore not related to the suspected pathophysiology of seizures. On the other hand, drugs for the acute treatment of seizures and status epilepticus (SE) are aimed at stopping seizures once they are occurring. These abortive drugs are somewhat mechanism-specific, and there is clinical value in reviewing the pathophysiology of generalized tonic-clonic seizures.

The basic premise of generalized tonic-clonic seizure pathophysiology is that seizures start with a robust excitation of susceptible epileptic cerebral neurons, which leads to synchronous discharges of progressively larger groups of connected neurons eventually affecting a part of the brain that leads to the clinical manifestations of the seizure. Although the inciting events are entirely unknown, it is clear that an imbalance of excess excitation and decreased inhibition sustains a seizure.[5] Glutamate is the most common excitatory neurotransmitter and mediates the excess excitation via the N-methyl-D-aspartate (NMDA) subtype receptor. This is undoubtedly of paramount importance and is the most logical site of action for antiseizure drugs. However, clinically useful NMDA antagonists have not had great success, probably because drugs affecting this system have other profound effects on learning and memory.

Gamma-aminobutyric acid (GABA) is the most common inhibitory neurotransmitter and is the site of action of many drugs used to abort seizures.[5] GABA neurotransmission via activation of the $GABA_A$ subtype receptor prevents neurons from excess excitation under normal circumstances. In some patients, GABA inhibition may be impaired and $GABA_A$-enhancing drugs restore the balance. Even when inhibition is not impaired at baseline, enhancing $GABA_A$ inhibition during a seizure or to prevent seizures is useful because it may overcome the excess excitation of a seizure. $GABA_A$-enhancing drugs, such as benzodiazepines, barbiturates, propofol, and some anesthetics, are highly effective at stopping seizures once they are in progress because they overwhelm the ongoing excitation. Unfortunately, they are not suitable long-term agents because patients often become tolerant to the inhibition-enhancing drug effect. This probably results from upregulation of GABA receptors or changes in receptor sensitivity.

SEIZURE AND EPILEPSY DEFINITIONS

The vocabulary of seizures and epilepsy is sometimes confusing with inexact labels, jargon, and arcane terminology that hinders communication.[6,7] At times definitions differ between not only patients and clinicians but also between reference works. The correct classification of seizures is important because the diagnostic strategy and treatment of seizures may vary with the type of seizure or epileptic syndrome.

Although clinicians know what constitutes a seizure, seizure definitions are often surprisingly inexact. The phrase, "The patient just had a seizure," usually describes a patient with a generalized tonic-clonic convulsion consisting of some abnormal motor movements followed by an alteration in consciousness. This operational use of "seizure" may or may not be correct, because other transient events that are best not thought of as seizures, such as syncope, may present with a similar clinical picture. As such, some basic definitions are in order.

Seizures are defined as finite episodes of disturbed cerebral function caused by abnormal, excessive, and synchronous electrical discharges in groups of cortical neurons. Various clinical phenomena may be apparent via observation, or the seizure may be subclinical and thus remain clinically inapparent.[7] Theoretically, any behavior or experience of cerebral function may represent seizure activity, but in practice only certain patterns frequently occur that allow for a classification schema.

Convulsion may be used clinically to refer to the motor manifestations of abnormal electrical activity and is synonymous with generalized motor seizures. *Nonconvulsive* seizure refers to seizure activity that does not involve motor symptomatology. *Tonic* refers to a sustained stiffening of muscles that commonly accompanies many seizures. *Clonic* means rhythmic movements or jerking of the muscles. Thus, *tonic-clonic* would accurately describe a convulsion with initial stiffening of the body and extremities followed by rhythmic contractions of muscle groups. *Aura* is commonly used to refer to any premonitory subjective symptoms or sensation that the patient experiences before a seizure. In actuality, an aura represents a focal seizure and a description of the aura may provide valuable localizing information of the area of the brain where the generalized seizure begins.[8]

Epilepsy refers to the clinical condition of a patient with recurrent, unprovoked seizures. It is not appropriately applied to seizures provoked by acute metabolic conditions or acute central nervous system (CNS) insults. For example, spontaneous recurrent seizures because of remote head injury or without an identifiable cause are deemed epilepsy, whereas a patient with seizures recurring only when provoked by hyponatremia or ethanol withdrawal are not considered to have epilepsy. *Seizure disorder* is synonymous with epilepsy; some use this term preferentially because of prejudicial associations with the term epilepsy.

SEIZURE ETIOLOGY AND CLASSIFICATION

Another component in the classification of seizures is their etiology. *Provoked seizures*, sometimes referred to as acute symptomatic seizures, are seizures from an identifiable cause such as electrolyte abnormalities, head injury, toxins, or infection. This is an important concept, because treatment of symptomatic seizures must take into consideration treatment not only of the seizure, but also of the underlying cause.

As mentioned previously, epilepsy is defined by recurrent spontaneous seizures for which no identifiable or provoking cause has been determined after investigation. *Post-ictal* refers to any of a variety of transient behaviors including alterations in consciousness that may follow a seizure. *Todd paralysis* refers to transient post-ictal paralysis that occurs in some patients, most commonly following a seizure that is confined to one hemisphere. *Anticonvulsant* is a term that refers to any medication used to treat seizures; this term has largely been replaced by the term *AEDs*.

At the bedside, the determination of the cortical origin of an observed behavior is largely conjectural. Assignment to the most likely seizure type is a preliminary step and likely to be revised as additional information becomes available. Recall that a differential diagnosis is necessary when determining the etiology of seizures, given that a variety of other events may occur suddenly, causing alteration in mental status or abnormal motor movements.[9] One initial diagnostic strategy is to divide transient phenomena or spells into seizures versus other types of spells. Seizures may be attributable to epilepsy or provoked in an otherwise healthy person as discussed previously. Spells that clinically resemble seizures to the casual, or even trained, observer are listed in **Box 1**. Syncope is often associated with bilateral tonic or clonic motor activity that looks exactly like a seizure but simultaneous electroencephalogram (EEG) recording reveals only severe suppression of brain activity rather than seizure discharges. Syncope is distinguished by the almost immediate return of normal consciousness, whereas generalized tonic-clonic seizures are always followed by a period of at least confusion, if not an unarousable state. Convulsive concussion is a similar phenomenon that can be observed during acute head trauma, as has been demonstrated during Australian football or rugby, in which motor activity resembling a seizure occurs on impact. Brainstem release phenomena can cause decerebrate or decorticate posturing, which is distinguished by the associated unresponsiveness and other clinical signs of brain injury. Movement disorders with involuntary movements may resemble seizures, but consciousness is always preserved in movement disorders. Young children can hold their breath long enough to decrease cerebral perfusion and cause syncope with associated motor movements, especially during a crying tantrum. Psychogenic nonepileptic spells are also termed pseudoseizures

---

Box 1
Differential diagnosis of seizures

1. Seizures: seizures from abnormal cortical discharge
   - Epilepsy (**Box 2**)
   - Provoked (acute symptomatic) seizures
2. Non-epileptic spells (NES): events that may resemble seizures in appearance but do not result from abnormal cortical electrical discharges
   - Convulsive syncope
   - Convulsive concussion
   - Repetitive decerebrate or decorticate posturing
   - Involuntary movement disorders
   - Breath-holding spells
   - Sleep disorders
   - Psychogenic nonepileptic spells (pseudoseizures)

because they resemble seizures but they are of psychiatric origin and the EEG is normal during the spell despite what is often wild thrashing. They have also been termed nonepileptic seizures, but again, this terminology is confusing because these events are not actually seizures resulting from excessive cortical activity.

A classification of seizure types based on that of the International League Against Epilepsy (ILAE) is the most widely used system.[7,10–12] Despite efforts to use such schemes to standardize defining seizure events, some interobserver variability has been noted in assignments to seizure types after reviewing historical information about the event.[13] A basic sorting distinction is to assign the seizure to that of a partial seizure or a generalized seizure (**Box 2**). When classifying a seizure as a partial seizure, it implies that the clinical information, including the history, observation, and EEG indicate that the initial cortical activation is limited to one part of one of the cerebral hemispheres. Partial seizures may further be classified into 3 groups: (1) simple partial seizures, (2) complex partial seizures, and (3) partial seizures secondarily generalized to involve the whole brain. This categorization scheme recognizes different symptoms of partial seizures by further dividing simple partial seizures into those with motor, sensory, or special sensory symptoms. The term *simple* partial seizure specifies seizures that do not cause an alteration in consciousness because they affect such a small part of the brain. The term *complex* is used to indicate seizures that include clouded or impaired

---

Box 2
Classification of clinical seizure types

Partial seizures

- Simple partial seizure
    1. Motor symptoms
    2. Sensory symptoms
    3. Special sensory symptoms
    4. Autonomic symptoms
    5. Psychic symptoms
- Complex partial seizure (consciousness is clouded)
    1. Simple partial onset followed by impaired consciousness
    2. Impairment of consciousness at onset
- Partial seizure evolving into generalized seizure

Generalized seizures

- Absence seizures
- Myoclonic seizures
- Clonic seizures
- Tonic seizures
- Tonic-clonic seizures
- Atonic seizures
- Others

Unclassifiable seizure types

Data from Refs.[2,5–7]

consciousness; the term *complex partial seizure* has largely replaced the older term, *psychomotor seizure.* Temporal lobe complex partial seizures, or temporal lobe seizures, typically begin with autonomic auras followed by a motionless stare or repetitive motor movements, such as chewing or finger picking.[7] If the electrical activity associated with a simple partial seizure or complex partial seizure spreads to involve both cerebral hemispheres, this indicates seizure evolution into a generalized seizure, manifested by symptoms consistent with bilateral cortical activity. This may occur too rapidly to be detectable by the clinicians, such that EEG monitoring or other clinical information may be required to establish the diagnosis. Partial seizures, either complex partial or secondarily generalized, are the most common seizure type in adults.

Seizures that represent initial bilateral cortical involvement are termed *generalized seizures.* This distinction is often made only following EEG monitoring and other clinical investigations that suggest that the seizure activity does not begin in one cortical area. Correct identification of partial or generalized seizures has implications for diagnosis and therapy. For example, a neurologically normal 2-year-old who experienced a brief generalized seizure might very well have had a simple febrile seizure; however, if that generalized seizure were preceded by a focal seizure, the differential diagnosis is significantly changed, as is the diagnostic workup and disposition because focal pathology is now suspected.

There are several types of generalized seizures. *Absence seizures,* previously termed *petit mal,* show a characteristic EEG pattern during the seizure (generalized typical 3-Hz spike and slow wave complexes) and are clinically manifested by brief staring episodes or an arrest in behavior. *Generalized tonic-clonic,* or *grand mal, seizures* are the most common of the generalized seizure types. Other generalized seizures types are *myoclonic* (brief, sudden muscular contractions), *clonic* (repetitive jerks without tonic phase), and *tonic* (rigid muscular contraction without rhythmic activity). *Atonic seizures* (loss of muscle tone) usually present with unprotected falling to the ground. Last, the organizational scheme allows for unclassified epileptic seizures, which include seizures that cannot be classified into one of the previously mentioned categories or those associated with incomplete data precluding classification.

STATUS EPILEPTICUS DEFINITIONS

SE has been generally defined as enduring seizure activity that is not likely to stop spontaneously. The traditional SE definition is 30 minutes of continuous seizure activity or 2 or more seizures without full recovery of consciousness between the seizures. There are as many types of SE as there are types of seizures. The distinction between convulsive and nonconvulsive SE depends on clinical observation and on a clear understanding of several SE types.[5,14]

Generalized convulsive SE (GCSE) is a medical emergency requiring prompt treatment. The need to urgently treat GCSE has prompted recent efforts to reduce the time requirement for seizure activity to only 5 minutes.[14] GCSE may involve seizures that are tonic-clonic, clonic, tonic, or myoclonic. GCSE may evolve as it persists over time, with a reduction in clinically apparent motor movements despite persistence in CNS seizure activity. Although this late stage of SE has been referred to as nonconvulsive SE, it is perhaps better labeled as end-stage, or *subtle SE.*[15]

Nonconvulsive SE encompasses enduring seizures that do not include generalized motor convulsions, such as absence SE or complex partial SE. The term nonconvulsive SE is best reserved for these epileptic twilight states, and should not be used for the subtle or transformed GCSE described previously (**Box 3**).

<table>
<tr><td>

Box 3
Classification of status epilepticus

Generalized convulsive status epilepticus

- Overt (convulsions obvious)
- Subtle (sometimes termed nonconvulsive status epilepticus or end-stage status)

Nonconvulsive status epilepticus

- Complex partial status epilepticus
- Absence (typical and atypical) status epilepticus
- Generalized nonconvulsive status epilepticus

Simple partial status epilepticus with motor symptoms

Other enduring seizure types

</td></tr>
</table>

EPILEPTIC SYNDROMES

Epileptic syndromes are used to condense clinical seizure information into meaningful groupings. If seizures are symptoms, and epilepsy is a disease, then there are some subsets of seizure disorders that may be made following correlation of clinical information and neurodiagnostic testing. These subsets are epilepsy syndromes and the correct assignment to a syndrome may help to convey clinical information. Unlike a seizure, a syndrome cannot be observed because it requires knowledge of data other than just the seizure type.[16] Assignment to an epilepsy syndrome is usually performed by the neurologist and is useful in that it may indicate some general thoughts about prognosis and expectations as well as being useful in clinical trials and other investigations. The final classification of seizure type or assignment to an epilepsy syndrome may follow neuroimaging, video recording, or EEG investigations, resources that are not available at the time of bedside observation. For the emergency physician, categorization of a patient to an epilepsy syndrome is not usually possible.

These epileptic syndromes can be thought of as specific disease entities with seizures representing a symptom of the disease. This is somewhat analogous to the clinical diagnosis of congestive heart failure (CHF); though CHF is a recognizable clinical picture with a general treatment pattern, it is ultimately a symptom of another disease process. In contradistinction to a disease, a syndrome does not necessarily have a common etiology and prognosis. However, identification of a specific epilepsy syndrome is essential to the diagnosis, treatment, and prognosis of patients with epilepsy.[16,17] The delineation and classification of epileptic syndromes is still ongoing, and many of the syndromes are uncommon or obscure.

Localization-related is used in epilepsy syndrome terminology instead of partial to indicate that seizures arise from pathology in a localizable area (**Table 1**).[2] Idiopathic, symptomatic, and cryptogenic categories are the other subdivisions. *Idiopathic* epilepsy syndromes do not have symptoms other than seizures and historically had no obvious underlying cause but it is becoming clear that most of the idiopathic syndromes are because of abnormalities of neurotransmission. Individuals with idiopathic epilepsy are usually otherwise neurologically normal. *Symptomatic* epilepsy syndromes imply that the seizures are "symptomatic" of underlying brain disease. *Cryptogenic* in this scheme refers to those disorders that are suspected to be symptomatic without definitive proof of an underlying cause and are referred to as *probably symptomatic epilepsy syndrome* in a proposed diagnostic scheme.[12]

Table 1
Classification of epileptic syndromes with examples

	Generalized (Named by Disease)	Localization-Related (Named by Location)
Idiopathic	Benign neonatal convulsions Childhood absence epilepsy Juvenile myoclonic epilepsy Epilepsy with generalized seizures Some reflex epilepsies Others	Benign childhood epilepsy with centro-temporal spikes Childhood epilepsy with occipital paroxysms Primary reading epilepsy
Symptomatic (known structural disease or etiology) or *Cryptogenic* (suspected but not demonstrable structural disease)	Cortical abnormalities • malformations • dysplasias Metabolic abnormalities • amino acidurias • organic acidurias • mitochondrial diseases • others West syndrome (infantile spasms) Lennox-Gastault syndrome Others	Temporal lobe • mesio-temporal lobe epilepsy • lateral temporal lobe epilepsy Frontal lobe • motor cortex • supplementary motor cortex • orbito-frontal • others Parietal lobe Occipital lobe Most reflex epilepsies

Data from Refs.[2,5–7,31]

West syndrome (age <1 year, infantile spasms, typical EEG pattern), Lennox-Gastaut syndrome (age 1–8 years, multiple seizure types, typical EEG pattern), and juvenile myoclonic epilepsy are examples of accepted epilepsy syndromes with specific age criteria, seizures types, clinical characteristics, or EEG findings. Some of the syndromes are commonly accepted, whereas others are less rigorously supported by evidence.[18] Even with initial detailed information, the diagnosis of epilepsy syndromes may change over time as more clinical information becomes available.[16,18,19] One organizational scheme of epilepsy syndromes classifies the epilepsies in tabular form, emphasizing the distinction between generalized and localization-related syndromes.[20]

ESSENTIAL QUESTIONS
Why Do Some Seizures Fail to Stop?

Some endogenous seizure-terminating process must exist or every seizure would persist. These processes are really unknown, but a variety of mechanisms have been postulated for seizure termination. The appearance of an abnormally prolonged seizure may be a manifestation of excessive excitation, a failure of inhibition, or a combination of the two processes. In the case of excitatory toxins, eg, cholinergic drug overdose, substances act directly on receptors to overexcite glutamate receptors. Failure of GABA inhibition during the course of a seizure may occur, leading to SE. In a chemically induced experimental model of GCSE, diazepam (a GABA receptor agonist) was less potent when administered later in the course of seizures than when given earlier.[21] This suggests that $GABA_A$ receptors may change in number or sensitivity during the course of SE. This concept is novel and has potential implications for treatment, as it implies that drugs that might be effective early in the course of status might not be effective later in the course. Experimental animal models suggest possible roles for some neuropeptides (neuropeptide Y, galanin) in seizure modulation.[22]

An unidentified genetic influence for SE has been suggested. A twin study found a concordance for epilepsy of 0.74 for monozygotic twins and 0.25 for dizygotic twins, but SE occurred in 3 of 13 monozygotic twin pairs and in none of 26 pairs of dizygotic twins.[23]

What Physiologic Changes Accompany Generalized Convulsive Status Epilepticus?

Striking physiologic changes accompany GCSE, largely reflecting the catecholamine surge that accompanies this condition. The physiologic responses are variable and conceptually it is useful to consider the responses in terms of "early" and "late." The consequences of GCSE can be thought of as a sequence of systemic, motor, and EEG events.[24] GCSE may lead to hyperthermia, leukocytosis, cerebrospinal fluid (CSF) pleocytosis, cardiovascular and respiratory abnormalities with lactic acidosis, serum glucose abnormalities, and elevation of serum catecholamines.[25,26] Cells in the CSF and hyperthermia are of course consistent with a possible CNS infection. Attributing these responses to SE is a process of exclusion and the possibility of an infectious etiology should always be considered. The acidosis produced from the muscular contractions of seizures may be striking but interventions other than actions to halt the convulsions are not needed; the lactic acidosis will be cleared quickly once the seizure stops.

An evolution of EEG changes that parallel physiologic changes has been proposed. Some of the seizures associated with generalized SE were observed to be focal or lateralized or fragments of a generalized convulsion. A proposed scheme envisions a sequence of motor and EEG changes in GCSE ranging from discrete motor and EEG events that merge into continuous seizures. The sequences evolve through episodic ictal discharges toward EEG findings of paroxysmal epileptiform discharges without accompanying motor activity. This final stage is essentially an electromechanical dissociation of brain electrical activity and motor activity.

Experimental GCSE in primates causes cellular damage in the neocortical, cerebellar, and hippocampal areas. When some of the systemic effects such as hypotension, muscle contractions, and respiratory depression were treated (paralyzed, ventilated animals) and other factors such as serum glucose were controlled, detectable brain injury still occurred in the hippocampus.[27] A summary of experimental work seems to confirm the concept that there are different stages of GCSE with early systemic changes being an elevation of blood pressure, serum glucose, and serum lactate. Brain metabolism is elevated but cerebral blood flow and substrate supply are adequate for demands. At some transition point between 30 and 60 minutes, irreversible neuronal injury starts, because of excitotoxic cell injury. Eventually, mismatch or decompensation occurs with brain metabolism remaining high but with cerebral blood flow and substrate supply declining (**Table 2**).[5]

In a review of hemodynamic monitoring in the day before death in patients in intensive care unit with SE, 2 patterns of mean arterial pressure (MAP) and heart rate (HR) were observed. One group showed a gradual decline in MAP and HR in the hours before death and was more likely to have cardiac risk factors, which were thought to result in progressive deterioration. The other group had acute cardiovascular deterioration without preceding decline in hemodynamic parameters, which the investigators speculated might be attributable to arrhythmias precipitated by GCSE.[28]

Table 2
Early and late phases of generalized convulsive status epilepticus

	Early Status Epilepticus (less than 30–60 minutes)	Late or Decompensated Status (more than 60 minutes)
Motor activity	Generalized convulsions	Fragmentary seizures, no convulsions
Electroencephalogram	Recurrent seizures	Continuous seizures then episodic
Blood pressure	Elevated	Decreased
Serum glucose	Elevated	Normal or decreased
Serum lactate	Elevated	Less elevated
Brain metabolism	Elevated	Elevated
Cerebral blood flow	Elevated	Decreased

Data from Lothman E. The biochemical basis and pathophysiology of status epilepticus. Neurology 1990;40(5 Suppl 2):13–23.

What Are the Consequences of Generalized Convulsive Status Epilepticus and Why Do They Occur?

GCSE is associated with a mortality of about 20% and the mortality of refractory GCSE is even higher.[25,29] Many of the deaths are associated with the underlying cause of the status. For example, refractory status associated with bacterial meningitis has a higher mortality than status associated with AED withdrawal or ethanol withdrawal. However, although a higher mortality is associated with GCSE, some types of status are not associated with a high mortality, eg, absence SE (3 cycle-per-second spike and wave activity; an epileptic twilight state). Likewise, enduring simple partial SE with motor symptoms (epilepsia partialis continua) is not associated with higher mortality or other morbidity.

In a study analyzing cause of death in patients with GCSE from diverse causes, duration of status for an hour or more was associated with increased mortality.[29] Anoxic damage and increasing age were associated with higher mortality, whereas seizure etiology of alcohol and AED withdrawal were associated with low mortality rates. Interestingly, in this study, the mortality rates of partial and generalized SE were not significantly different; the investigators suspected that the combination of focal brain injury and partial SE contributed to the high mortality.[29]

Clinically there are events accompanying GCSE that are associated with increased mortality. A marker for CNS injury has been sought for some years. Neuron-specific enolase, an enzyme important for energy metabolism in the brain, is elevated both in serum and CSF after generalized SE. The neuronal injury is thought to allow the enzyme to leak out, presumably through membrane damage. Blood-brain-barrier disruption is suspected to be a factor as well. Interestingly, increased neuron-specific enolase has also been demonstrated to be elevated following complex partial SE as well suggesting that cellular damage occurred with this type of nonconvulsive status. The elevations of neuron-specific enolase following complex partial and other nonconvulsive SE is somewhat surprising because clinically this entity is not thought to be injurious or approached as aggressively as GCSE. It was suggested that high levels of neuron-specific enolase reflect the long duration of complex partial SE. Subclinical SE (subtle SE, end-stage SE) was associated with the highest levels of neuron-specific enolase thought to be reflecting the severity of the neurologic injury in that group.[30] The neurologic injury is thought to result primarily from the excessive abnormal neuronal discharges and not from the physiologic changes that accompany status alone.

Excitotoxic mechanisms are probably the most important mediator of neuronal injury in SE (**Fig. 1**).[5] When glutamate binds to the NMDA subtype of glutamate receptors under normal circumstances, nothing happens because the channel is blocked by a large magnesium ion stuck in the pore. However, under the severely depolarized conditions of SE, the magnesium ion is no longer held in the pore and the channel is not occluded. This allows calcium and other ions to flow into the neuron. Because of the unusual properties of this channel, it does not close but instead is further activated by this influx of calcium. This leads to the pathologic accumulation of intracellular calcium, causing intracellular havoc. Neurons die by acute necrosis from this insult and by activation of second messenger mechanisms that lead to delayed cell death or apoptosis.

Experimental GCSE causes morphologic damage in the hippocampal area in animal models with a pattern of neuronal cell loss and gliosis equivalent to mesial temporal sclerosis seen in many patients with temporal lobe epilepsy. Experimental GCSE also causes axonal reactions (mossy fiber sprouting) also found in human temporal lobe epilepsy.[3,22] The simple idea that "seizures beget seizures" implies that SE may predispose patients to additional seizures in the future and gives credence to aggressive measures to terminate GCSE.

FUTURE DIRECTIONS

Continued progress with basic research may affect treatment of seizures and SE in the emergency department. Current thoughts of pathophysiology of GCSE suggest that aggressive prompt termination of GCSE may positively affect patient outcomes. New formulations of existing drugs, such as intranasal administration of benzodiazepines, and new parenteral drugs to abort seizures will be available in the near future and will change treatment strategies. New neuroprotective drugs that prevent neuronal injury

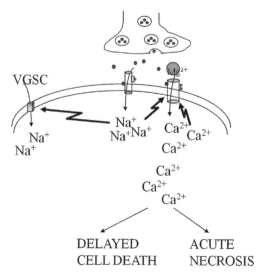

Fig. 1. NMDA-mediated excitotoxicity.

even if they do not stop seizure activity, such as NMDA antagonists, may become available. New EEG technologies may influence treatment in the emergency department by detecting subtle SE and guiding treatments.

SUMMARY

Seizures result from recurrent excitatory connections in the cerebral cortex and a loss of synchronization between aggregates of neurons. Seizures produce a number of physiologic consequences, and if seizures are prolonged, homeostatic mechanisms deteriorate. Animal models suggest that even if systemic factors such as acidosis and hypoxia are controlled, prolonged SE results in neuronal damage from neurotoxic amino acids and calcium influx. It appears that SE alone may result in cognitive impairment and epileptogenesis regardless of the inciting cause. GCSE is present when as little as 5 minutes of continuous seizure activity occurs.

Clinical communications will be improved with a correct classification of seizure types. The basic distinction in seizure types is that of generalized and partial seizures. Nonepileptic spells include psychogenic seizures but also may include convulsive syncope and other transient events that are not of cortical electrical origin.

KEY CONCEPTS

- Seizures are thought to occur from a variety of pathophysiological mechanisms that are incompletely understood.
- Failures of inhibitory processes are thought to be responsible for the failure of many seizures to terminate spontaneously.
- Status epilepticus injures the brain directly through prolonged abnormal electrical activity.
- Five minutes of continuous convulsive seizure activity defines generalized convulsive status epilepticus
- Correct seizure terminology improves clinical communications and may affect therapy

---

REFERENCES

1. Mulley JC, Scheffer IE, Petrou S, et al. Channelopathies as a genetic cause of epilepsy. Curr Opin Neurol 2003;16(2):171–6.
2. Steinlein OK, Mulley JC, Propping P, et al. A missense mutation in the neuronal nicotinic acetylcholine receptor alpha 4 subunit is associated with autosomal dominant nocturnal frontal lobe epilepsy. Nat Genet 1995;11(2):201–3.
3. Sutula T, Cascino G, Cavazos J, et al. Mossy fiber synaptic reorganization in the epileptic human temporal lobe. Ann Neurol 1989;26(3):321–30.
4. Andermann F. Cortical dysplasias and epilepsy: a review of the architectonic, clinical, and seizure patterns. Adv Neurol 2000;84:479–96.
5. Fountain NB, Lothman EW. Pathophysiology of status epilepticus. J Clin Neurophysiol 1995;12(4):326–42.
6. Dasheiff RM. The unbearable quaintness of neurology. JAMA 1989;262(1):30.
7. Mosewich RK, So EL. A clinical approach to the classification of seizures and epileptic syndromes. Mayo Clin Proc 1996;71(4):405–14.
8. Luders HO, Burgess R, Noachtar S. Expanding the international classification of seizures to provide localization information. Neurology 1993;43(9):1650–5.
9. Morrell MJ. Differential diagnosis of seizures. Neurol Clin 1993;11(4):737–54.

10. Proposal for revised classification of epilepsies and epileptic syndromes. Commission on Classification and Terminology of the International League Against Epilepsy. Epilepsia 1989;30(4):389–99.
11. Proposal for revised clinical and electroencephalographic classification of epileptic seizures. From the Commission on Classification and Terminology of the International League Against Epilepsy. Epilepsia 1981;22(4):489–501.
12. Engel J Jr. A proposed diagnostic scheme for people with epileptic seizures and with epilepsy: report of the ILAE Task Force on Classification and Terminology. Epilepsia 2001;42(6):796–803.
13. Bodensteiner JB, Brownsworth RD, Knapik JR, et al. Interobserver variability in the ILAE classification of seizures in childhood. Epilepsia 1988;29(2):123–8.
14. Lowenstein DH, Bleck T, Macdonald RL. It's time to revise the definition of status epilepticus. Epilepsia 1999;40(1):120–2.
15. Treiman DM, Meyers PD, Walton NY, et al. A comparison of four treatments for generalized convulsive status epilepticus. Veterans Affairs Status Epilepticus Cooperative Study Group. N Engl J Med 1998;339(12):792–8.
16. Benbadis SR, Luders HO. Epileptic syndromes: an underutilized concept. Epilepsia 1996;37(11):1029–34.
17. Berg AT, Shinnar S, Levy SR, et al. Newly diagnosed epilepsy in children: presentation at diagnosis. Epilepsia 1999;40(4):445–52.
18. Berg AT, Shinnar S, Levy SR, et al. How well can epilepsy syndromes be identified at diagnosis? A reassessment 2 years after initial diagnosis. Epilepsia 2000; 41(10):1269–75.
19. Camfield P, Camfield C. Childhood epilepsy: what is the evidence for what we think and what we do? J Child Neurol 2003;18(4):272–87.
20. Benbadis SR. Epileptic seizures and syndromes. Neurol Clin 2001;19(2):251–70.
21. Kapur J, Macdonald RL. Rapid seizure-induced reduction of benzodiazepine and Zn2+ sensitivity of hippocampal dentate granule cell GABAA receptors. J Neurosci 1997;17(19):7532–40.
22. Kapur J. Status epilepticus in epileptogenesis. Curr Opin Neurol 1999;12(2): 191–5.
23. Corey LA, Pellock JM, Boggs JG, et al. Evidence for a genetic predisposition for status epilepticus. Neurology 1998;50(2):558–60.
24. Lothman E. The biochemical basis and pathophysiology of status epilepticus. Neurology 1990;40(5 Suppl 2):13–23.
25. Aminoff MJ, Simon RP. Status epilepticus. Causes, clinical features and consequences in 98 patients. Am J Med 1980;69(5):657–66.
26. Simon RP. Physiologic consequences of status epilepticus. Epilepsia 1985; 26(Suppl 1):S58–66.
27. Blennow G, Brierley JB, Meldrum BS, et al. Epileptic brain damage: the role of systemic factors that modify cerebral energy metabolism. Brain 1978;101(4): 687–700.
28. Boggs JG, Marmarou A, Agnew JP, et al. Hemodynamic monitoring prior to and at the time of death in status epilepticus. Epilepsy Res 1998;31(3):199–209.
29. Towne AR, Pellock JM, Ko D, et al. Determinants of mortality in status epilepticus. Epilepsia 1994;35(1):27–34.
30. DeGiorgio CM, Heck CN, Rabinowicz AL, et al. Serum neuron-specific enolase in the major subtypes of status epilepticus. Neurology 1999;52(4):746–9.
31. Fountain NB. Manual of antiepileptic drug therapy. West Islip(NY): Professional Publications Inc; 2010.

Emergency Department Seizure Epidemiology

Jennifer L. Martindale, MD[a,b,c,d,e],
Joshua N. Goldstein, MD, PhD[c,d,e], Daniel J. Pallin, MD, MPH[a,b,c,e],*

KEYWORDS

- Seizure • Acute symptomatic seizure • Epilepsy
- Status epilepticus • Epidemiology

Etymologically, both "seizure" and "epilepsy" refer to a removal of the victim from reality. The patient is "seized up," or "taken hold of" (the Greek *lepsis* connotes *taking hold of* or *grasping*). Seizure is an *ictus*, or sudden event, comprising a pathologic pattern of cortical activity resulting in abnormal involuntary movement or change in consciousness. Seizures are categorized broadly as unprovoked, acute symptomatic (secondary to an acute insult), childhood febrile, and psychogenic. Epilepsy is defined by the occurrence of at least 2 unprovoked seizures.

Seizure is a common problem in emergency medicine, accounting for about 1 of every 100 emergency department (ED) visits in the United States.[1] The epidemiology of epilepsy has been studied well, but less has been written about the epidemiology of seizures in patients who do not have epilepsy.[1–5] A systematic review of the literature identified 25 original research articles describing ED seizure patients.[1,6–29] Among these, 3 analyzed data from more than 1000 patients.[1,15,27] One prospective study included 1833 seizure patients who had neuroimaging at 11 university-affiliated United States EDs from July 1996 to September 1998; patients aged 5 years or younger were excluded.[15] Another included 1011 ED seizure patients, but its generalizability was limited by the fact that it excluded seizures caused by alcohol and drugs, medication-related hypoglycemia, recent trauma, and epilepsy.[27] The most recent and

[a] Department of Emergency Medicine, Brigham and Women's Hospital, 75 Francis Street, Boston, MA 02115, USA
[b] Division of Emergency Medicine, Children's Hospital, 300 Longwood Avenue, Boston, MA 02115, USA
[c] Harvard-Affiliated Emergency Medicine Residency, 75 Francis House, Neville House, 236A, Boston, MA 02115, USA
[d] Department of Emergency Medicine, Massachusetts General Hospital, 55 Fruit Street, Boston, MA 02114, USA
[e] Harvard Medical School, Boston, MA, USA
* Corresponding author. 75 Francis Street, Boston, MA 02115.
E-mail address: dpallin@partners.org

Emerg Med Clin N Am 29 (2011) 15–27
doi:10.1016/j.emc.2010.08.002
0733-8627/11/$ – see front matter © 2011 Elsevier Inc. All rights reserved.

emed.theclinics.com

largest descriptive study analyzed a systematic sample of all United States ED visits from 1993 to 2003 from the National Hospital Ambulatory Medical Care Survey.[1] In this study, 3215 seizure-related visits were identified and national estimates calculated. One informative study was conducted outside the ED setting,[2] and included all acute symptomatic seizures that came to medical attention in Rochester, Minnesota, from 1955 to 1984.

EPIDEMIOLOGY OF SEIZURES IN THE ED SETTING

About 11% of people in the United States will have one or more seizures during their lifetime, most of which are not due to epilepsy.[3] The most common type of seizure is the pediatric febrile seizure, affecting about 4% of the population; by definition the occurrence of the febrile seizure is limited to ages 6 months to 6 years.[30] By age 80, 3.6% of people in the United States will suffer at least one acute symptomatic seizure (not including febrile seizures).[2] Epilepsy is diagnosed at some point in life in 3% of people in the United States.[3]

Gender

Males account for a greater proportion of seizures in the ED setting, with an odds ratio of 1.4 for the association between male gender and seizure among ED visits in the United States.[1] On a population level (rather than in the ED setting), acute symptomatic seizures occur in males versus females in a ratio of 1.85 to 1, with a lifetime risk of 5.0% in males and 2.7% in females.[2] By contrast, epilepsy is only slightly more common in males.[31] The increased incidence of acute symptomatic seizures in males is not due to alcohol or trauma, as the male predominance persists across all etiologic categories except toxic, eclamptic, and metabolic seizures.[2]

Race

Among United States ED visits for seizure, African Americans are overrepresented relative to Caucasians, with an odds ratio of 1.4.[1] Moreover, African American ED seizure patients are less likely to receive neuroimaging than Caucasians, with an odds ratio of 0.6.[1]

Age

Seizure of any type is most likely after age 75 years, due to stroke and other cumulative causes of structural brain damage.[2] Acute symptomatic seizures, in contrast, have a bimodal age distribution (**Table 1**).[2] The incidence is highest among infants, at 253 per 100,000, followed by those aged greater than or equal to 75, at 123 per 100,000.[2] The lowest incidence is among those 25 to 34 years old, at 15 per 100,000.

Children aged 1 to 5 years account for more ED visits for seizure than any other age group, followed by adults aged 41 to 50 (**Fig. 1**).[1] The high occurrence among small children is a result of the febrile seizure, accounting for 28% of all pediatric ED seizures.[21] The high rate among those aged 41 to 50 is multifactorial, due only in part to ethanol-related seizures.[1]

Among children, after infancy, first time afebrile seizures are most common at school age, and all afebrile seizures (first time and otherwise) increase with age because of the cumulative prevalence of epilepsy.[22]

ETIOLOGY OF SEIZURE IN THE ED

Most seizures managed in the ED are secondary to an underlying disease process, that is, they are either acute symptomatic seizures or pediatric febrile seizures.

Table 1	
Population-based epidemiology of acute symptomatic seizures	
Age Group	**Seizures per 100,000 Person-Years Observation**
<1	252.9
1–4	42.1
5–14	18.4
15–24	20.1
25–34	15.4
35–44	27.0
45–54	43.6
55–64	55.0
65–74	82.3
75+	123.2
All ages	39.0

Data from Annegers JF, Hauser WA, Lee JR, et al. Incidence of acute symptomatic seizures in Rochester, Minnesota, 1935–1984. Epilepsia 1995;36(4):327–33.

In a nationwide study of United States ED visits for seizure, 66% had at least one diagnosis in addition to seizure.[1] The most common codiagnoses were alcohol related, followed by otitis media (likely relevant due to febrile seizures) and hypertension.

Another descriptive study of ED patients analyzed 1833 ED seizure patients who had neuroimaging.[15] A prior seizure history was documented in 44%. Seizure types were: generalized (86%), focal motor (6.2%), partial complex (4.7%), and unknown (3.1%). Diagnoses were available for 1348 of the cases, and are displayed in **Fig. 2**. The 3 most common causes were alcohol and drugs (19%), head injury (7.8%), and epilepsy (6.8%), though the cause was not reported or was reported as "unknown" or "other" in 48.8% of cases. Neurocysticercosis was the etiological factor in 9% of Hispanic ED seizure patients.

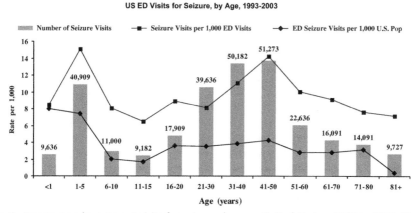

Fig. 1. Emergency department visits for seizure, by age, United States, 1993 to 2003. (*From* Pallin DJ, Goldstein JN, Moussally JS, et al. Seizure visits in US emergency departments: epidemiology and potential disparities in care. Int J Emerg Med 2008;1(2):101; with permission from Springer Science+Business Media.)

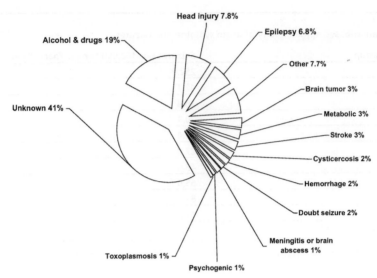

Head injury 7.8%

Epilepsy 6.8%

Alcohol & drugs 19%

Other 7.7%

Brain tumor 3%

Unknown 41%

Metabolic 3%

Stroke 3%

Cysticercosis 2%

Hemorrhage 2%

Doubt seizure 2%

Meningitis or brain
abscess 1%

Toxoplasmosis 1%

Psychogenic 1%

Fig. 2. Causes of all seizures among patients older than 5 years who had neuroimaging at 11 university-affiliated EDs, United States, July 1996 to September 1998. (*From* Ong S, Talan DA, Moran GJ, et al. Neurocysticercosis in radiographically imaged seizure patients in U.S. emergency departments. Emerg Infect Dis 2002;8(6):610; with permission.)

The contribution of "breakthrough seizures" among chronic epileptics to the burden of seizure care in the ED setting is unknown. The aforementioned study[15] suggested that only 6.8% of seizures in the ED were due to epilepsy. However, a smaller study in a different setting found that 46% of seizure visits to an urban ED were by known epileptics.[10]

A study by Annegers and colleagues[2] provided the etiologic breakdown (**Fig. 3**) of acute symptomatic seizures for an entire population (not in the ED setting). Although small ED series have found few seizure patients with metabolic abnormalities, large ED series have found that 2.9% to 5% of seizures result from metabolic causes, not including hypoxia.[15,27]

Ethanol withdrawal was diagnosed as the cause of up to 28% of seizures in the studies reviewed.[17] Alcohol withdrawal does not account for all seizures related to alcohol abuse. In one study, withdrawal could explain only 22% of the seizures attributed to alcohol abuse.[10] Alcohol-related seizures can be caused by metabolic derangement, cerebral disorders, other drug abuse, trauma, and latent epilepsy unmasked by alcohol. Whether alcohol can cause seizure by direct toxic effect on neurons remains controversial.[32] A case-control study of alcohol use and seizure suggested that "seizures can be interpreted as a disorder induced by the ingestion of alcohol, independently of alcohol withdrawal."[33]

Among children the febrile seizure is most common, accounting for almost a third of pediatric ED seizures.[21] Febrile seizures in children are classified as simple versus complex (focal, duration >15 minutes, or more than once in 24 hours).[30] About 20% of first febrile seizures are complex.[34]

In babies younger than 6 months, an important role for hyponatremia was established by Farrar and colleagues.[7] In 47 infants younger than 6 months "who lacked other findings suggesting a cause," hyponatremia was thought to be the cause of seizure in 70%.

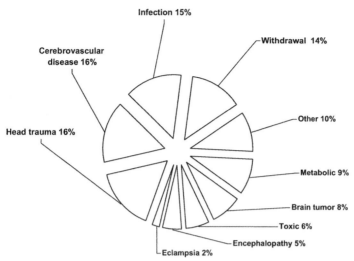

Fig. 3. Causes of acute symptomatic seizures in the entire population of Rochester, Minnesota, 1955 to 1984. (*From* Annegers JF, Hauser WA, Lee JR, et al. Incidence of acute symptomatic seizures in Rochester, Minnesota, 1935–1984. Epilepsia 1995;36(4):327–33; with permission.)

Trauma is an important cause of seizures. Immediate posttraumatic seizures are uncommon, and their significance unclear. The Canadian Head CT Study excluded patients who seized after their trauma, and the New Orleans study found seizure to be a reason to proceed with head computed tomography (CT).[35,36] In one large Chinese series, 2.4% of patients with mild head trauma seized within a week of their trauma (including both immediate posttraumatic seizures and later seizures); 47% of these had an intracranial traumatic abnormality on CT, and 7% had surgical craniotomies.[37] Chronic epilepsy is often due to head trauma.[38] Trauma also occurs as a result of seizure.[10,39]

Many diseases have presented as seizures in the ED, for example, pheochromocytoma,[40] postpartum eclampsia,[41] misuse of phosphate-containing enemas causing hypocalcemia,[42] and child abuse with water intoxication causing hyponatremia.[43] Very rarely, ionic and nonionic contrast myelography, common outpatient procedures, can cause seizures.[44,45] Cerebrospinal fluid shunt malfunction may present as seizure, though only 2.9% of seizure episodes in shunted children lead to shunt revision.[46]

Differential Diagnostic Considerations

Clinical presentations of other acute illnesses can mimic seizure and vice versa. In one study of 166 children presenting with a chief complaint of seizure, 110 (66%) had a different diagnosis.[12] Cardiac arrhythmia, asystole, myocardial infarction, and myocarditis are causes of both real seizures and seizure-like presentations in all age groups.[47–52]

Seizures can also present in atypical ways. Seizure can cause acute pulmonary edema.[53,54] Seizure might be the cause of syncope in 29% to 53% of patients older than 15 years, and 7.5% of younger patients.[55,56] Seizures can present as bizarre forms of altered mental status, or cause isolated aphasia masquerading as stroke.[57–60]

Few acute seizures are attributable to meningitis. Green and colleagues[61] reviewed 503 pediatric meningitis cases and found that 115 had seizures prior to the diagnosis of meningitis. No case of bacterial meningitis presented solely with fever and seizure; all children with meningitis were obtunded, had nuchal rigidity, had prolonged focal seizures, or had multiple seizures and a petechial rash. The investigators concluded that seizure in febrile children does not mandate lumbar puncture. Partially treated meningitis, like all partially treated infections, represents a special diagnostic dilemma.[62] Children who survive meningitis are at increased risk for epilepsy (4.2% overall, 6% for *Haemophilus influenzae*, and 14% for pneumococcus).[63] Although many patients with bacterial meningitis have seizures,[61,62,64] the number of patients with seizure who have bacterial meningitis is unknown and probably extremely small, and lumbar puncture is not considered a routine diagnostic test among afebrile immunocompetent seizure patients.

SEIZURE EPIDEMIOLOGY IN THE PREHOSPITAL SETTING

Seizure patients are more likely to be transported by ambulance than other patients, and certain states may mandate that paramedics be dispatched for management and advanced life support transport of patients with seizure. In one study, 54% of ED seizure patients arrived by ambulance.[10] Seizures account for 5.6% to 9% of pediatric Emergency Medical Services transports.[65-68] Seizures were the reason for transport in 1.7% of patients aged 60 years or older in a semi-urban North Carolina county.[69] New Mexico investigators studied seizure as a factor in repeated ambulance use. In the Albuquerque area, with "approximately 40,000" ambulance transports per year, seizure was the seventh most common chief complaint.[70] From 1992 to 1994, there were 3383 transports of 2319 seizure patients (about 3% of all transports), with the highest per-patient transport number being 39.[70]

McArthur and Rooke[71] reviewed all patients transported to an urban ED for a 10.5-year period to determine the frequency of spinal injury in uncomplicated seizure patients. Of 1656 cases, there were no spinal injuries. Spinal precautions resulted in a 113% increase in transportation costs and a 57% increase in nursing costs. One study suggested that seizure patients requiring advanced life support care can be identified by advanced responders at the scene, and triage to basic life support transport was unlikely to result in a bad outcome.[65]

SEIZURE RECURRENCE AND PROGNOSIS

Epileptologists have found that 35% to 40% of patients with a first-time unprovoked seizure will have a recurrence within 2 years.[4] However, it is important to remember that unprovoked seizures and recurrent unprovoked seizures (ie, "epilepsy") constitute only a small minority of the seizures seen in the ED.[15] In a cohort of patients followed for 10 years after presenting to an ED for an acute symptomatic seizure (excluding children with febrile seizure), 13% went on to have an unprovoked seizure.[29] This risk was significantly greater (41%) for those patients who had acute symptomatic status epilepticus. Most occurred within 2 years of the first seizure.

Simple febrile seizures are a normal part of childhood, and have an excellent prognosis. The risk of recurrence is high, and ranges from about 12% in children whose first febrile seizure occurs in infancy to about 50% in those whose first febrile seizure occurs later.[9,42] The subsequent risk of epilepsy is the same as for children who have never had a febrile seizure. Complex febrile seizures, on the other hand, do indicate an increased risk for epilepsy, and do not indicate an increased risk for future occurrence of simple febrile seizure.[5]

Disposition

A quarter of ED seizure visits end in hospital admission.[1] Patients more likely to be admitted are older, have received neuroimaging, and have a high-risk codiagnosis, such as alcohol withdrawal, pneumonia, cerebrovascular disease, hypoglycemia, septicemia, hypokalemia, brain neoplasm, or intracranial injury. In a multicenter study of 368 patients 23% of all seizure patients were admitted, versus 63% of first-time seizure patients.[8]

STATUS EPILEPTICUS

Status epilepticus is defined as 30 minutes or more of seizure, or of multiple seizures with failure to regain consciousness between them. In ED-based series, when status was mentioned, it represented 6% to 7% of seizures.[8,10,28] In 1995, DeLorenzo and colleagues[72] estimated 195,000 status events in 152,000 patients per year in the United States, with 42,000 deaths. The highest rate was in infants, followed by the elderly. Fewer than half of the cases were managed by neurologists, and the majority (58%) occurred in patients with no prior history of epilepsy. Overall mortality was 22%, with an age-related increase from 3% in children to 38% in the elderly. Whites were affected less frequently (23 per 100,000) than nonwhites (71 per 100,000), but mortality in whites was 31% versus 17% in nonwhites. In adults, risk factors were: low antiepileptic drug levels (34%), remote insults (24%), stroke (22%), metabolic derangement (15%), ethanol (13%), hypoxia (13%), infection, tumor, anoxia, central nervous system infection, trauma, and idiopathic. In children, risk factors were: infection (52%), remote insult (39%), low antiepileptic drug levels (21%), stroke, metabolic, hypoxia, idiopathic, trauma, and ethanol.

Nonconvulsive status is electrical status without predominant motor activity. Whether it is very harmful is a subject of debate.[73–75] It accounts for about a quarter of status episodes, and has been observed to persist in 48% of cases after control of convulsive status.[76,77] Nonconvulsive status has been found in 8% of comatose patients, leading some neurologists to recommend screening for occult status epilepticus among patients in coma of unclear etiology.[78]

PSYCHOGENIC SEIZURES

Psychogenic seizures are reported to account for 20% of patients at epilepsy referral centers, and up to 50% of patients with refractory status epilepticus.[79,80] Estimates put the prevalence of psychogenic seizures in the general population at 30 per 100,000, comparable to multiple sclerosis and more common than Guillan-Barré.[81] In one study, 24% of patients with recurrent psychogenic seizures had the onset attributed to a head injury.[82] Efforts to stop psychogenic seizures have caused significant morbidity.[79,83–86] Diagnosis of psychogenic seizures is often delayed (>7 years in one German cohort of 313 patients).[87]

COST AND BURDEN OF DISEASE ATTRIBUTABLE TO SEIZURE IN THE ED SETTING

Robust estimates of the cost of ED seizure care are not available, but several lines of evidence suggest the magnitude of the problem. Seizures account for about 1% of ED visits nationwide, and about 2% of visits to children's hospital EDs.[1,8,21,25,43] In a Canadian series,[88] 13.8% of ED seizure patients suffered injury and 1.2% died;

the estimated annual population incidence for injury or death among patients seen in the ED for seizure was 32.2 per 100,000. Population-based studies in Rochester, Minnesota have found the cumulative lifetime incidence of epilepsy to be 3%, of all unprovoked seizures 4%, and of any convulsive disorder 11%.[3] The World Health Organization estimated in 2000 that 0.5% of the total global burden of disease is attributable to epilepsy alone (not including febrile seizures and acute symptomatic seizures, which affect more people than epileptic seizures).[89]

A national study estimated the number of seizure-related visits to United States EDs at approximately 1 million per year, during 1993 to 2003.[1] The median cost of an ED visit was estimated in 2007 to be $498.[90] If it is assumed that the mean cost of an ED visit for seizure to be close to this median figure, and that costs have risen since 2007, one can estimate that over half a billion dollars are spent annually for ED seizure care. The cost of prehospital care is also significant. The average cost of an ambulance ride estimated in 2004 was $415, and about half of ED seizure patients arrive by ambulance.[10,91] Given 1 million United States ED visits for seizure annually, this suggests annual expenditures for prehospital care of seizure patients on the order of $200 million. These rough estimates are not adjusted for inflation. More robust estimation would require primary research to ascertain the costs and variability of ED and prehospital seizure care. It seems reasonable, nonetheless, to conclude that the cost of prehospital and ED care of seizure patients in the United States is close to $1 billion annually.

SUMMARY

Seizures account for about 1% of ED visits nationwide, and about 2% of visits to children's hospital EDs. Males are overrepresented among ED patients with seizure, and not just due to gender differences in trauma or substance abuse. The costs of ED and prehospital seizure care are unknown, but the authors estimate that they are on the order of $1 billion annually in the United States.

Status epilepticus occurs in about 6% of ED seizure patients; most cases occur in patients without a known seizure disorder. Status has an overall mortality rate of 22%, with an age-related increase from 3% in children to 38% in the elderly. Psychogenic seizures are about as common in the general population as multiple sclerosis, and up to half of cases of refractory status epilepticus may be psychogenic.

The best available evidence suggests that most seizures among ED patients are unrelated to epilepsy, except in older children. Seizing infants may have hyponatremia. In young children febrile seizures are most common. In adults and the elderly, alcohol and vascular causes predominate, but a host of other conditions may cause seizure.

Many questions remain to be answered regarding the epidemiology of seizures in emergency medicine. Why are seizures so much more common in males? What are the outcomes for patients seen in the ED with seizure? How do outcomes depend on demographic predictors, such as age and race, versus underlying etiology? To what extent do seizures continue to be confused with other disease states?

Epilepsy is the purview of the neurologist, but it is the emergency physician who is charged with elucidating the epidemiology of nonepileptic seizures, which constitute the bulk of seizures managed in the ED setting.

ACKNOWLEDGMENTS

Many thanks to Andy Jagoda, and to Alex Green and Jon Moussally for comments on the manuscript.

KEY CONCEPTS

- Seizure accounts for 1 of every 100 ED visits in the United States, and about 1 in 50 visits in United States Children's hospital EDs.

- The pediatric febrile seizure occurs from 6 months to 6 years of age, and is common and benign, affecting 4% of children.

- Psychogenic seizures are an important consideration, especially in refractory status epilepticus.

- First-time seizure causes vary widely, and include hyponatremia in infants younger than 6 months, epilepsy in older children, alcoholism in adults, and vascular disease in the elderly.

- The cost of ED seizure care is unknown, but is likely to be on the order of $1 billion per year in the United States.

REFERENCES

1. Pallin DJ, Goldstein JN, Moussally JS, et al. Seizure visits in US emergency departments: epidemiology and potential disparities in care. Int J Emerg Med 2008;1(2):97–105.
2. Annegers JF, Hauser WA, Lee JR, et al. Incidence of acute symptomatic seizures in Rochester, Minnesota, 1935–1984. Epilepsia 1995;36(4):327–33.
3. Hauser WA, Annegers JF, Rocca WA. Descriptive epidemiology of epilepsy: contributions of population-based studies from Rochester, Minnesota. Mayo Clin Proc 1996;71(6):576–86.
4. Berg AT, Testa FM, Levy SR, et al. The epidemiology of epilepsy. Past, present, and future. Neurol Clin 1996;14(2):383–98.
5. Berg AT. Febrile seizures and epilepsy: the contributions of epidemiology. Paediatr Perinat Epidemiol 1992;6(2):145–52.
6. Eisner RF, Turnbull TL, Howes DS, et al. Efficacy of a "standard" seizure workup in the emergency department. Ann Emerg Med 1986;15(1):33–9.
7. Farrar HC, Chande VT, Fitzpatrick DF, et al. Hyponatremia as the cause of seizures in infants: a retrospective analysis of incidence, severity, and clinical predictors. Ann Emerg Med 1995;26(1):42–8.
8. Huff JS, Morris DL, Kothari RU, et al. Emergency department management of patients with seizures: a multicenter study. Acad Emerg Med 2001;8(6):622–8.
9. Kenney RD, Taylor JA. Absence of serum chemistry abnormalities in pediatric patients presenting with seizures. Pediatr Emerg Care 1992;8(2):65–6.
10. Krumholz A, Grufferman S, Orr ST, et al. Seizures and seizure care in an emergency department. Epilepsia 1989;30(2):175–81.
11. Earnest MP, Feldman H, Marx JA, et al. Intracranial lesions shown by CT scans in 259 cases of first alcohol-related seizures. Neurology 1988;38(10):1561–5.
12. Landfish N, Gieron-Korthals M, Weibley RE, et al. New onset childhood seizures. Emergency department experience. J Fla Med Assoc 1992;79(10):697–700.
13. McKee PJ, Wilson EA, Dawson JA, et al. Managing seizures in the casualty department. BMJ 1990;300(6730):978–9.
14. Nypaver MM, Reynolds SL, Tanz RR, et al. Emergency department laboratory evaluation of children with seizures: dogma or dilemma? Pediatr Emerg Care 1992;8(1):13–6.
15. Ong S, Talan DA, Moran GJ, et al. Neurocysticercosis in radiographically imaged seizure patients in U.S. emergency departments. Emerg Infect Dis 2002;8(6):608–13.

16. Powers RD. Serum chemistry abnormalities in adult patients with seizures. Ann Emerg Med 1985;14(5):416–20.

17. Rosenthal RH, Heim ML, Waeckerle JF. First time major motor seizures in an emergency department. Ann Emerg Med 1980;9(5):242–5.

18. Scarfone RJ, Pond K, Thompson K, et al. Utility of laboratory testing for infants with seizures. Pediatr Emerg Care 2000;16(5):309–12.

19. Schoenenberger RA, Heim SM. Indication for computed tomography of the brain in patients with first uncomplicated generalised seizure. BMJ 1994;309(6960): 986–9.

20. Sempere AP, Villaverde FJ, Martinez-Menendez B, et al. First seizure in adults: a prospective study from the emergency department. Acta Neurol Scand 1992; 86(2):134–8.

21. Sharma S, Riviello JJ, Harper MB, et al. The role of emergent neuroimaging in children with new-onset afebrile seizures. Pediatrics 2003;111(1):1–5.

22. Shinnar S, O'Dell C, Mitnick R, et al. Neuroimaging abnormalities in children with an apparent first unprovoked seizure. Epilepsy Res 2001;43(3):261–9.

23. Tardy B, Lafond P, Convers P, et al. Adult first generalized seizure: etiology, biological tests, EEG, CT scan, in an ED. Am J Emerg Med 1995;13(1):1–5.

24. Turnbull TL, Vanden Hoek TL, Howes DS, et al. Utility of laboratory studies in the emergency department patient with a new-onset seizure. Ann Emerg Med 1990; 19(4):373–7.

25. Choquet C, Depret-Vassal J, Doumenc B, et al. Predictors of early seizure recurrence in patients admitted for seizures in the Emergency Department. Eur J Emerg Med 2008;15(5):261–7.

26. Farhidvash F, Singh P, Abou-Khalil B, et al. Patients visiting the emergency room for seizures: insurance status and clinic follow-up. Seizure 2009;18(9): 644–7.

27. Henneman PL, DeRoos F, Lewis RJ. Determining the need for admission in patients with new-onset seizures. Ann Emerg Med 1994;24(6):1108–14.

28. Brinar V, Bozicevic D, Zurak N, et al. Epileptic seizures as a symptom of various neurological diseases. Neurol Croat 1991;40(2):93–101.

29. Hesdorffer DC, Logroscino G, Cascino G, et al. Risk of unprovoked seizure after acute symptomatic seizure: effect of status epilepticus. Ann Neurol 1998;44(6): 908–12.

30. Steering Committee on Quality Improvement and Management, Subcommittee on Febrile Seizures American Academy of Pediatrics. Febrile seizures: clinical practice guideline for the long-term management of the child with simple febrile seizures. Pediatrics 2008;121(6):1281–6.

31. Kotsopoulos IA, van Merode T, Kessels FG, et al. Systematic review and meta-analysis of incidence studies of epilepsy and unprovoked seizures. Epilepsia 2002;43(11):1402–9.

32. Bartolomei F, Suchet L, Barrie M, et al. Alcoholic epilepsy: a unified and dynamic classification. Eur Neurol 1997;37(1):13–7.

33. Ng SK, Hauser WA, Brust JC, et al. Alcohol consumption and withdrawal in new-onset seizures. N Engl J Med 1988;319(11):666–73.

34. Verity CM, Golding J. Risk of epilepsy after febrile convulsions: a national cohort study. BMJ 1991;303(6814):1373–6.

35. Haydel MJ, Preston CA, Mills TJ, et al. Indications for computed tomography in patients with minor head injury. N Engl J Med 2000;343(2):100–5.

36. Stiell IG, Wells GA, Vandemheen K, et al. The Canadian CT head rule for patients with minor head injury. Lancet 2001;357(9266):1391–6.

37. Lee ST, Lui TN. Early seizures after mild closed head injury. J Neurosurg 1992; 76(3):435–9.
38. Annegers JF, Hauser WA, Coan SP, et al. A population-based study of seizures after traumatic brain injuries. N Engl J Med 1998;338(1):20–4.
39. Desai BT, Whitman S, Coonley-Hoganson R, et al. Seizures in relation to head injury. Ann Emerg Med 1983;12(9):543–6.
40. Leiba A, Bar-Dayan Y, Leker RR, et al. Seizures as a presenting symptom of phaeochromocytoma in a young soldier. J Hum Hypertens 2003;17(1):73–5.
41. D'Addesio JP. Postpartum eclampsia. Ann Emerg Med 1989;18(10):1105–6.
42. Walton DM, Thomas DC, Aly HZ, et al. Morbid hypocalcemia associated with phosphate enema in a six-week-old infant. Pediatrics 2000;106(3):E37.
43. Tilelli JA, Ophoven JP. Hyponatremic seizures as a presenting symptom of child abuse. Forensic Sci Int 1986;30(2–3):213–7.
44. Dunford J. Fatal ascending tonic-clonic seizure syndrome. Ann Emerg Med 1998; 32(5):624–6.
45. Olsen J. Seizures after myelography with Iopamidol. Am J Emerg Med 1994; 12(3):329–30.
46. Johnson DL, Conry J, O'Donnell R. Epileptic seizure as a sign of cerebrospinal fluid shunt malfunction. Pediatr Neurosurg 1996;24(5):223–7 [discussion: 227–8].
47. Smith-Demps C, Jagoda A. A case of seizure-related bradycardia and asystole. Am J Emerg Med 1998;16(6):582–4.
48. Cunningham R, Silbergleit R. Viral myocarditis presenting with seizure and electrocardiographic findings of acute myocardial infarction in a 14-month-old child. Ann Emerg Med 2000;35(6):618–22.
49. Herman LL, Stoshak M, Rittenberry TJ. Long QT syndrome presenting as a seizure. Am J Emerg Med 1992;10(5):435–8.
50. Linzer M, Grubb BP, Ho S, et al. Cardiovascular causes of loss of consciousness in patients with presumed epilepsy: a cause of the increased sudden death rate in people with epilepsy? Am J Med 1994;96(2):146–54.
51. Moller JC, Ballnus S, Kohl M, et al. Evaluation of the performance of general emergency physicians in pediatric emergencies: obstructive airway diseases, seizures, and trauma. Pediatr Emerg Care 2002;18(6):424–8.
52. Venkataraman V, Wheless JW, Willmore LJ, et al. Idiopathic cardiac asystole presenting as an intractable adult onset partial seizure disorder. Seizure 2001; 10(5):359–64.
53. Brambrink AM, Tzanova I. Neurogenic pulmonary oedema after generalized epileptic seizure. Eur J Emerg Med 1998;5(1):59–66.
54. Darnell JC, Jay SJ. Recurrent postictal pulmonary edema: a case report and review of the literature. Epilepsia 1982;23(1):71–83.
55. Martikainen K, Seppa K, Viita P, et al. Transient loss of consciousness as reason for admission to primary health care emergency room. Scand J Prim Health Care 2003;21(1):61–4.
56. Pratt JL, Fleisher GR. Syncope in children and adolescents. Pediatr Emerg Care 1989;5(2):80–2.
57. Garmel GM, Jacobs AK, Eilers MA. Tonic status epilepticus: an unusual presentation of unresponsiveness. Ann Emerg Med 1992;21(2):223–7.
58. Glassman JN, Dryer D, McCartney JR. Complex partial status epilepticus presenting as gelastic seizures: a case report. Gen Hosp Psychiatry 1986;8(1):61–4.
59. LaCapra S, King C. Mute postseizure patient: an unusual manifestation of Todd's phenomenon. Ann Emerg Med 1994;23(4):877–80.
60. Soslow AR. Psychomotor seizures. Ann Emerg Med 1984;13(4):290–2.

61. Green SM, Rothrock SG, Clem KJ, et al. Can seizures be the sole manifestation of meningitis in febrile children? Pediatrics 1993;92(4):527–34.
62. Rosenberg NM, Meert K, Marino D, et al. Seizures associated with meningitis. Pediatr Emerg Care 1992;8(2):67–9.
63. Baraff LJ, Lee SI, Schriger DL. Outcomes of bacterial meningitis in children: a meta-analysis. Pediatr Infect Dis J 1993;12(5):389–94.
64. Cabellos C, Verdaguer R, Olmo M, et al. Community-acquired bacterial meningitis in elderly patients: experience over 30 years. Medicine (Baltimore) 2009;88(2):115–9.
65. Abarbanell NR. Prehospital seizure management: triage criteria for the advanced life support rescue team. Am J Emerg Med 1993;11(3):210–2.
66. Johnston C, King WD. Pediatric prehospital care in a southern regional emergency medical service system. South Med J 1988;81(12):1473–6.
67. Knight S, Vernon DD, Fines RJ, et al. Prehospital emergency care for children at school and nonschool locations. Pediatrics 1999;103(6):e81.
68. Tsai A, Kallsen G. Epidemiology of pediatric prehospital care. Ann Emerg Med 1987;16(3):284–92.
69. Wofford JL, Moran WP, Heuser MD, et al. Emergency medical transport of the elderly: a population-based study. Am J Emerg Med 1995;13(3):297–300.
70. Brokaw J, Olson L, Fullerton L, et al. Repeated ambulance use by patients with acute alcohol intoxication, seizure disorder, and respiratory illness. Am J Emerg Med 1998;16(2):141–4.
71. McArthur CL 3rd, Rooke CT. Are spinal precautions necessary in all seizure patients? Am J Emerg Med 1995;13(5):512–3.
72. DeLorenzo RJ, Hauser WA, Towne AR, et al. A prospective, population-based epidemiologic study of status epilepticus in Richmond, Virginia. Neurology 1996;46(4):1029–35.
73. Drislane FW. Evidence against permanent neurologic damage from nonconvulsive status epilepticus. J Clin Neurophysiol 1999;16(4):323–31.
74. Kaplan PW. No, some types of nonconvulsive status epilepticus cause little permanent neurologic sequelae (or: "the cure may be worse than the disease"). Neurophysiol Clin 2000;30(6):377–82.
75. Krumholz A, Sung GY, Fisher RS, et al. Complex partial status epilepticus accompanied by serious morbidity and mortality. Neurology 1995;45(8):1499–504.
76. DeLorenzo RJ, Waterhouse EJ, Towne AR, et al. Persistent nonconvulsive status epilepticus after the control of convulsive status epilepticus. Epilepsia 1998; 39(8):833–40.
77. Drislane FW. Presentation, evaluation, and treatment of nonconvulsive status epilepticus. Epilepsy Behav 2000;1(5):301–14.
78. Towne AR, Waterhouse EJ, Boggs JG, et al. Prevalence of nonconvulsive status epilepticus in comatose patients. Neurology 2000;54(2):340–5.
79. Howell SJ, Owen L, Chadwick DW. Pseudostatus epilepticus. Q J Med 1989; 71(266):507–19.
80. Lesser RP. Psychogenic seizures. Neurology 1996;46(6):1499–507.
81. Benbadis SR, Allen Hauser W. An estimate of the prevalence of psychogenic non-epileptic seizures. Seizure 2000;9(4):280–1.
82. Barry E, Krumholz A, Bergey GK, et al. Nonepileptic posttraumatic seizures. Epilepsia 1998;39(4):427–31.
83. Bateman DE. Pseudostatus epilepticus. Lancet 1989;2(8674):1278–9.
84. Gunatilake SB, De Silva HJ, Ranasinghe G. Twenty-seven venous cutdowns to treat pseudostatus epilepticus. Seizure 1997;6(1):71–2.

85. Reuber M, Baker GA, Gill R, et al. Failure to recognize psychogenic nonepileptic seizures may cause death. Neurology 2004;62(5):834–5.
86. Smith PE, Saunders J, Dawson A, et al. Intractable seizures in pregnancy. Lancet 1999;354(9189):1522.
87. Reuber M, Fernández G, Bauer J, et al. Diagnostic delay in psychogenic nonepileptic seizures. Neurology 2002;58(3):493–5.
88. Kirby S, Sadler RM. Injury and death as a result of seizures. Epilepsia 1995;36(1): 25–8.
89. Available at: http://www.who.int/whr2001/2001/archives/2000/en/pdf/Annex4-en. pdf. Accessed August 30, 2003.
90. Table 6: Emergency Room Services-Median and Mean Expenses per Person With Expense and Distribution of Expenses by Source of Payment: United States, 2007. Medical Expenditure Panel Survey. Agency for Health Research and Quality, US Department of Health and Human Services. Available at: http:// www.meps.ahrq.gov/exchweb/bin/redir.asp?URL=https://phsexchweb.partners.org/ exchweb/bin/redir.asp?URL=http://www.meps.ahrq.gov/. Accessed August 13, 2010.
91. Ambulance providers: costs and expected Medicare margins vary greatly GAO-07-383. GAO US Government and Accountability Office. Available at: http://www. gao.gov/new.items/d07383.pdf. Accessed August 14, 2010.

The Diagnosis and Management of Seizures and Status Epilepticus in the Prehospital Setting

Glen E. Michael, MD, Robert E. O'Connor, MD, MPH*

KEYWORDS

• Seizure • Prehospital seizure management • Status epilepticus
• Emergency medical services

Generalized tonic-clonic convulsions are the most common and dramatic type of seizure prompting calls to 911.[1–4] Patients who experience a seizure but do not have a known seizure disorder challenge the prehospital provider in identifying an underlying cause for the event. Patients with seizures who are otherwise back to normal are at risk for recurrent seizures and would likely benefit from hospital evaluation. Seizures typically terminate spontaneously in less than 5 minutes, but when protracted seizures represent a true medical emergency. Treatment of status epilepticus with benzodiazepines in the prehospital setting has the potential to dramatically affect patient outcomes.[5,6] In all cases, the cornerstone of sound transport and treatment is sound Emergency Medical Services (EMS) system medical oversight. This article discusses the current controversies surrounding the prehospital evaluation and management of patients presenting to EMS with seizure.

INCIDENCE OF SEIZURES IN THE PREHOSPITAL SETTING

In a review of 87,203 calls received by a 911 center in Cleveland, Ohio, 3967 (5%) had a chief complaint of "convulsions" or "seizure."[1] A retrospective review of ambulance run reports for patients younger than 18 years from the Birmingham Regional Emergency Medical Service System indicated that approximately 8% of all pediatric calls were for seizure, a proportion slightly higher than in the adult population.[2] In a multistate analysis of pediatric EMS transports, seizures were among the 3 most common medical complaints identified.[3] Frequent interventions included oxygen administration,

Department of Emergency Medicine, University of Virginia School of Medicine, PO Box 800699, Charlottesville, VA 22908, USA
* Corresponding author.
E-mail address: reo4x@virginia.edu

Emerg Med Clin N Am 29 (2011) 29–39
doi:10.1016/j.emc.2010.08.003
0733-8627/11/$ – see front matter © 2011 Elsevier Inc. All rights reserved.

intravenous access, and administration of medications. The frequency of complaints relating to seizure in the prehospital setting underscores the need for training of EMS personnel on its diagnosis and management.

PREHOSPITAL SEIZURE EVALUATION AND MANAGEMENT

Prehospital management of seizures typically begins with a call to 911 whereby EMS dispatchers can gather vital information to guide prehospital management. Key background information includes bystander assessment of airway, breathing, and pulse. The dispatcher should then verify whether the patient is still actively seizing, then ask if there is any history of cardiac problems, prior seizures, pregnancy, diabetes, trauma, or overdose.[4]

If time permits, emergency medical technicians (EMTs) should obtain additional history from bystanders, such as whether the seizure started with an aura or was focal in nature. The EMTs should also attempt to determine whether the patient has a history of seizures, is taking anticonvulsants, and if he or she has been compliant in taking medications.

Most seizures will have stopped before EMS arrival. If not, status epilepticus is likely. Whether the seizure is ongoing or not, proper care of the patient begins with an assessment of airway, breathing, and circulation. Suction should be available and supplemental oxygen should be given. EMTs must anticipate the need for bag-valve-mask assisted ventilation if cyanosis is present, the respiratory rate is slow, or respiratory effort is poor. Patients with seizures frequently require intravenous (IV) access for medications. Although obtaining prehospital IV access has been shown to prolong scene time in seizure patients, having an IV in place is extremely helpful should the patient have another seizure and is usually justified.[7,8]

Seizure patients should receive supportive care during transport, including attention to identification of treatable causes such as hypoxia and hypoglycemia (**Boxes 1–3**). Patients with a history of diabetes requiring medications should not routinely receive glucose empirically, but should await the performance of a point-of-care glucose determination.

Spinal precautions are not routinely necessary in all seizure patients. A 1995 retrospective chart review spanning a 10-year period was conducted to evaluate the incidence of spinal injury in uncomplicated seizure patients.[9] A total of 1656 seizure cases were reviewed, and no spinal injuries were found. Transportation costs increased approximately 113% and nursing costs increased approximately 57% for patients with seizures placed in spinal precautions. The investigators concluded that eliminating the need for spinal precautions in seizure patients would result in significant cost savings without increased morbidity.

Patient refusal of EMS treatment and transport is an important consideration in prehospital seizure management. EMS providers must ascertain whether the patient wishing to refuse care has the capacity for medical decision making. An estimated 3% to 10% of base physician contacts by prehospital care providers are for patient-initiated refusal of care.[10,11] Such patients must demonstrate to providers the mental capacity to make an informed medical decision to refuse care. In patients who have just had a seizure, it is unlikely that they will demonstrate intact mental status and capacity for medical decision making.[12,13] Because the risk of seizure recurrence is approximately 6%, prehospital care providers and medical command physicians should ensure that patients understand the risks of refusal.[14]

Pediatric patients present unique challenges in prehospital seizure management. Galustyan and colleagues[15] studied the care of 1516 pediatric EMS calls with a chief

---

Box 1
Suggested paramedic orders for general patient care

- Perform scene survey
- Observe universal precautions
- Consider the need for additional resources
- Determine responsiveness
- Evaluate airway, breathing, circulation, and disability, exposing the patient as necessary
- Secure a patent airway as needed
- Manage cervical spine as needed
- Treat life-threatening conditions
- Monitor patient via the use of pulse oximetry and/or capnography, as appropriate
- Administer oxygen as appropriate (maintain an SaO_2 of at least 92%)
- For patients younger than 12 years, use length-based measurements to estimate equipment size and drug dosages
- Obtain medical history (history of present illness, past medical history, allergies, and medications)
- Evaluate blood pressure, pulses, respiratory rate, and temperature. Reassess with a frequency indicated by patient condition
- Monitor cardiac rhythm (12-lead electrocardiograph as appropriate)
- Assign treatment priority and make transport decision
- Establish intravenous access as appropriate
- Contact medical oversight for additional orders if needed
- Transport patient to the nearest appropriate medical facility without delay. Transport should be made safely and in a manner as to prevent further injury through the appropriate use of lights and sirens
- Transfer care of the patient to an appropriately trained health care provider

---

complaint of seizure. Of those calls, 189 (17%) refused transport. A history of seizure disorder was reported in 782 subjects (52%), of whom 598 (76%) were on chronic anti-convulsant therapy. A total of 390 subjects (26%) required treatment with benzodiazepines because of ongoing seizure activity. Of the 288 subjects who received diazepam by EMS, 79 (11%) were new-onset seizures.

Box 2
Suggested paramedic orders for adult seizure protocol (Active)

- Determine serum blood glucose by glucometer and administer up to 25 g dextrose 50% (D_{50}) if the blood glucose is less than 80 mg/dL
- Administer up to 2 mg midazolam (Versed) intravenously (slowly) if the patient continues to have generalized seizures. If unable to obtain intravenous access, 2 mg midazolam should be given intramuscularly. These doses may be repeated if seizures persist
- Administer 5 g magnesium sulfate intravenously over 10 minutes for seizures secondary to eclampsia

---

Box 3
Suggested paramedic orders for pediatric seizures (Active)

- If blood sugar is less than 80 mg/dL via glucometer, administer IV/intraosseous (IO) dextrose at the following dose and dilution (maximum dose 25 g):

    Dextrose 50% (D_{50}) at 1.0 mL/kg for children older than 2 years

    Dextrose 25% (D_{25}) at 2.0 mL/kg for children younger than 2 years

    Dextrose 12.5% ($D_{12.5}$) at 4.0 mL/kg for neonates

- Administer 0.2 mg/kg midazolam (Versed) up to a maximum dose of 5 mg IV, IO, or intramuscularly (IM) for seizure activity greater than 5 minutes in duration

---

Prehospital management of the patient who is actively seizing should also focus on the primary survey with anticipatory airway management. In generalized seizures, the gag reflex is suppressed and vomiting may result in aspiration of gastric contents. The patient should therefore be placed in a left lateral decubitus position and, when applicable, have his or her dentures removed. Due to risk to rescuers, a bite block should not be placed if the patient is actively seizing. Oropharyngeal airways pose risks similar to bite blocks. If an airway adjunct is necessary to support assisted ventilation during an active seizure, a nasopharyngeal airway is a safer alternative. It should be obvious (but worth the reminder) that rescuers should never put their fingers in the patient's mouth during a seizure, as jaw muscle spasms can cause serious bite injuries.

If the seizure was not witnessed, EMS providers should attempt to gather information that can help hospital personnel determine its cause. Witnesses should be queried regarding the duration of the seizure; specific seizure activity, such as eye deviation, bladder or bowel incontinence, mental status, and tonic-clonic muscle movements; events leading up to the seizure, including history of fever, trauma, or substance use; and whether multiple seizures occurred, either at this time or on a previous occasion. Additional history that should be elicited from bystanders includes whether the seizure started with an aura, whether it was focal in nature, whether the patient is on any antiepileptic drugs, and whether the patient has been compliant with those medications.

SEIZURE AND STATUS EPILEPTICUS MANAGEMENT IN CHILDREN

The classical definition of status epilepticus is a single seizure lasting continuously for more than 30 minutes, or 2 or more seizures with no recovery of normal mental status and function in between episodes. The operational definition of status epilepticus for EMS should be simplified, and includes any seizure that continues from the time 911 is called until EMS arrives on the scene, or any patient who remains postictal on EMS arrival and then experiences another event.

Diazepam is administered to patients in generalized convulsive status epilepticus (GCSE) by paramedics in many EMS systems throughout the United States. Alldredge and colleagues[16] reviewed the clinical course of GCSE in children to determine the effect of prehospital diazepam therapy (given rectally or intravenously). Nineteen patients were treated with prehospital diazepam; 9 with rectal diazepam (mean dose: 0.6 mg/kg) and 10 with IV diazepam (mean dose: 0.2 mg/kg). Twenty patients received no parenteral therapy and served as controls. Prehospital diazepam was associated with GCSE of shorter duration (32 minutes vs 60 minutes) and a reduced likelihood of recurrent seizures in the emergency department (ED) (58% vs 85%).

There were no significant differences between rectal and intravenous diazepam therapy with regard to duration of status epilepticus, intubation, or recurrent seizures in the ED. These data suggest that prehospital administration of diazepam may shorten the duration of GCSE in children and simplify the subsequent management of these patients in the ED.[17]

Galustyan and colleagues[15] performed a retrospective review of short-term outcomes comparing 2 emergency medical service treatment protocols in children 0 to 18 years old with seizure activity. During the control period, the EMS protocol recommended a diazepam dose of 0.2 to 0.5 mg/kg IV or per rectum (PR) for termination of seizure activity. During the intervention period, the diazepam dose was reduced to 0.05 to 0.1 mg/kg IV or PR. A total of 1516 subjects met the enrollment criteria: 1003 (66%) in the high-dose group and 513 (34%) in the reduced-dose group. EMS administered diazepam to 288 subjects: 189 (19%) in the high-dose group and 99 (19%) in the reduced-dose group. Subjects in the high-dose group were 9.7 times more likely to require intubation (19 patients in the high-dose group [10%], 1 patient in the reduced-dose group [1%]). Mean diazepam dose actually given was 0.17 mg/kg in the high-dose group and 0.13 mg/kg in the reduced-dose group (mean difference 0.04). No significant difference in the requirement for repeated anticonvulsant dose, complications, or ED interventions were noted. Hospital admission rate was lower in the reduced-dose group. This study demonstrated a reduction in intubation rate and need for hospitalization in the reduced diazepam dose EMS protocol. The reduction in the diazepam dose was effective at terminating seizure activity and did not increase the risk of adverse events.

In another study on prehospital seizure management in children, diazepam was compared with midazolam.[18] A retrospective review of the medical records of children presenting with seizures requiring treatment in the field by paramedics was performed over a 4-year period. In the EMS system studied, children with seizures were given 0.5 mg/kg PR or 0.1 mg/kg IV diazepam during the control period, and 0.15 mg/kg intramuscularly (IM) or 0.1 mg/kg IV midazolam during the investigational period. The main outcome measured was cessation of seizure. Secondary outcomes included time taken to initiate treatment and the frequency of cardiopulmonary compromise. Over the 4-year period, 2566 children presented with a seizure and 107 children (4%) were eligible for entry into the study. Of these 107 patients, 62 received diazepam and 45 received midazolam. Both groups were similar in terms of demographics and seizure type. A comparison of diazepam with midazolam showed that both drugs were effective in stopping seizures within 5 minutes of drug administration. A similar retrospective study comparing prehospital diazepam to midazolam was conducted more recently, and produced comparable results showing no significant difference in rates of seizure termination, seizure recurrence in the ED, airway intervention, or hospital admission between the diazepam and midazolam groups.[19]

Chamberlain and colleagues[20] compared treatment of ongoing seizures using IM midazolam versus IV diazepam. Children with generalized seizures of more than 10 minutes' duration were randomized to one of the two groups, and time to cessation of seizures was recorded. Twenty-four patients were enrolled (13 midazolam, 11 diazepam). Initial treatment with either midazolam or diazepam was successful in 22 of the 24 patients. One patient in each group failed therapy, and eventually required endotracheal intubation and general anesthesia for convulsive status epilepticus lasting more than 1 hour. Patients in the midazolam group received medication sooner (3.0 minutes vs 7.8 minutes) and had more rapid cessation of their seizures (7.8 minutes vs 11.2 minutes) than patients randomized to receive diazepam. The investigators concluded that IM midazolam is an effective anticonvulsant for children with motor seizures. Compared with IV diazepam, IM midazolam resulted in more rapid cessation of seizures because of more rapid administration. The IM route of administration may be particularly useful in the prehospital setting, owing to difficulty in quickly establishing IV access.

Vilke and colleagues[21] assessed the effectiveness and safety of IV and IM midazolam in the treatment of pediatric seizures by paramedics. Midazolam was administered to 74 patients with 49 IV doses and 25 IM doses. Improvement was reported for 91% (67/74) of patients. Greater success was reported with IV drug administration (47/49, 96%) than with IM administration (20/25, 80%). The investigators concluded that prehospital IV and IM midazolam are both effective interventions for pediatric seizures, but that IV administration is more effective.

Intranasal midazolam has been proposed as another potential therapy that may be conducive to the prehospital management of pediatric seizures. In a study comparing intranasal midazolam to rectal diazepam in a pediatric EMS population, Holsti and colleagues[22] found that intranasal midazolam was more effective at terminating seizures, was associated with fewer respiratory complications, and resulted in fewer hospital admissions as compared with rectal diazepam. In this study of 124 pediatric patients with seizure activity witnessed by EMS, 39 patients receiving intranasal midazolam were compared with 18 patients receiving rectal diazepam. Median seizure time witnessed by EMS was significantly longer for the diazepam group than for the midazolam group (30 minutes vs 11 minutes, $P = .003$). Children in the rectal diazepam group were more likely to experience a recurrent seizure in the ED (odds ratio [OR] 8.4, 95% confidence interval [CI] 1.6–43.6), require intubation in the ED (OR 12.2, 95% CI 2.0–75.4), and require hospitalization (OR 29.3, 95% CI 3.0–288.6).

SEIZURE AND STATUS EPILEPTICUS MANAGEMENT IN ADULTS

To determine whether the administration of benzodiazepines by paramedics is an effective and safe treatment for out-of-hospital status epilepticus, Alldredge and colleagues[5] conducted a randomized, double-blind trial comparing intravenous diazepam (5 mg), lorazepam (2 mg), and placebo. The Prehospital Treatment of Status Epilepticus (PHTSE) study was designed to address the following aims: (1) to determine whether administration of benzodiazepines by paramedics is an effective and safe means of treating status epilepticus in the prehospital setting and whether this therapy influences longer-term patient outcome, (2) to determine whether lorazepam is superior to diazepam for the treatment of status epilepticus in the prehospital setting, and (3) to determine whether control of status epilepticus before arrival to the ED influences patient disposition.

Adults with prolonged (lasting 5 minutes or more) or repetitive generalized convulsive seizures were eligible. Of the 205 patients enrolled, 66 received lorazepam, 68 received diazepam, and 71 received placebo. Status epilepticus was more likely to be terminated by the time of arrival to the ED in patients treated with lorazepam (59.1%) or diazepam (42.6%) compared with patients given placebo (21.1%) ($P = .001$). After adjustment for covariates, the odds ratio for termination of GCSE by the time of arrival in the lorazepam group as compared with the placebo group was 4.8 (95% CI 1.9–13.0). The odds ratio when comparing diazepam to placebo was 2.3 (95% CI 1.0–5.9). No statistically significant difference was found when directly comparing the lorazepam and diazepam groups (OR 1.9, 95% CI 0.8–4.4) The rates of respiratory or circulatory complications after the study treatment was administered were 10.6% for the lorazepam group, 10.3% for the diazepam group, and 22.5% for the placebo group ($P = .08$). The investigators concluded that benzodiazepines are safe and effective when administered by paramedics for out-of-hospital status epilepticus in adults. It was also concluded that lorazepam is likely to be a better therapy than diazepam.

Intravenous access cannot always be obtained rapidly when treating status epilepticus outside the hospital. Two studies conducted in an outpatient (non-EMS) setting compared the efficacy and safety of diazepam rectal gel to IV lorazepam in adults with seizures.[23,24] Rectal diazepam significantly reduced the likelihood of seizure recurrence during an episode of acute repetitive seizures, with minimal safety concerns. In addition, diazepam rectal gel was given more quickly and reliably, reducing total seizure time, potential neuronal injury, and other complications.

Kuisma and Roine[25] studied the safety and efficacy of intravenous propofol in the out-of-hospital treatment of convulsive status epilepticus in 8 patients. Convulsions ceased promptly after patients received a bolus of 100 to 200 mg propofol administered in the prehospital setting. The median duration of coma was 3 hours 15 minutes (range 2–41 hours), and the median duration of hospital treatment was 3.5 days (range 12 hours to 23 days). No adverse effects were observed except for a transient decrease in systolic blood pressure. Additional studies may be needed to verify this preliminary study, which seems to indicate that propofol is a potentially useful drug for the prehospital treatment of recurrent seizures refractory to standard management.

Fosphenytoin and parenteral valproate may prove useful for the prehospital management of GCSE. Advantages of fosphenytoin over phenytoin include more convenient and rapid intravenous administration, availability for intramuscular injection, and lower potential for adverse local reactions at injection sites. The rapid achievement of effective circulating concentrations permits the use of fosphenytoin in emergency situations, such as GCSE. Following intramuscular administration, therapeutic phenytoin plasma concentrations are observed within 30 minutes and maximum plasma concentrations occur at approximately 30 minutes for fosphenytoin and at 2 to 4 hours for derived phenytoin.[26] The Food and Drug Administration (FDA) has approved parenteral valproate for use in rapid loading and when oral therapy is impossible. Valproate has a broad spectrum of efficacy and may be useful in patients with absence or myoclonic status epilepticus. Adverse effects include local irritation, gastrointestinal distress, and lethargy. This drug is not FDA-approved for the treatment of status epilepticus.[27]

TRIAGE CONSIDERATIONS

There has been one study investigating triage criteria for advanced life support (ALS) versus non-ALS transport when faced with the seizure patient.[28] Preselected triage criteria for acuity of care based on neurologic condition, vital signs, and concomitant illness or injury were tested against retrospective data (paramedic run reports) collected on 230 patients. In 57 of these cases, need for ALS intervention was established on initial patient assessment. Of 173 patients requiring no ALS intervention on initial assessment, only 1 (0.58%) developed complications warranting ALS therapy during the course of prehospital care. The data presented in this study suggest that in urban settings with similar field times, after initial patient assessment by ALS personnel it is reasonable and safe to triage seizure patients who do not require ALS intervention to non-ALS rescue teams for continuation of care and transportation.

Hoffman and colleagues[29] reviewed written and audio records of paramedic-base hospital radio contact to determine whether care differed from that suggested in standard prehospital care protocols. Records of 659 contacts for seizure, syncope, abdominal pain, or altered mental state (28.4% of all EMS contacts) were scored for the use of standard therapies (such as intravenous access, oxygen, or naloxone) and unanticipated therapies (intubation, nitroglycerin). Cases that involved unanticipated treatments were reviewed to determine whether they could have been prospectively identified by simple clinical findings. Standard therapies were used in the majority of patients. Unanticipated therapies were administered to 13 patients, all of whom had abnormal vital signs, diaphoresis, respiratory distress, or a second prominent symptom. These data suggest that standard protocols could replace radio contact for most patients and that the few who might benefit from radio contact can be easily identified. The resulting reduction in need for on-line medical direction could produce significant cost savings.

Several studies have attempted to determine whether prehospital dispatch protocols, such as the Medical Priority Dispatch System (MPDS), can predict the need for ALS intervention based solely on information obtained at the time of an initial 911 call.[30–32] With regard to seizures, Shah and colleagues[30] found that even those patients assigned the lowest acuity category based on MPDS dispatch criteria required ALS interventions in 46% of cases. Sporer and colleagues[31] found that the low-acuity MPDS seizure group required treatment with midazolam in 7% of cases. With these high rates of time-dependent ALS interventions in even the low-acuity seizure category, the investigators concluded that all 911 calls for seizure should receive an initial ALS response.

COMPLICATIONS

GCSE is a medical emergency with a high morbidity and mortality rate. Reported mortality rates range from 15% to 37% in adults and from 3% to 15% in children, with a trend toward higher death rates in patients older than 65, in patients without a previous history of epilepsy, and in episodes lasting more than 1 hour.[33–35] Acute complications result from hyperthermia, pulmonary edema, cardiac arrhythmias, and cardiovascular collapse. Long-term complications include chronic seizure disorder (20%–40%), encephalopathy (6%–15%), and focal neurologic deficits (9%–11%).[34]

Other medical complications of status epilepticus include anoxia, cardiac rhythm disturbances, hypertension or hypotension, apnea, neurogenic pulmonary edema and congestion, aspiration pneumonia, airway, renal failure, fluid and electrolyte loss, metabolic acidosis, hyperkalemia, hyponatremia, hypoglycemia, hepatic failure, disseminated intravascular coagulation, hyperthermia, decreased cerebral perfusion, permanent neurologic dysfunction, worsened seizure state, and death.

FUTURE DIRECTIONS

Although prehospital seizure management has been relatively well studied, there remains ample opportunity for further inquiry in this field. A large, multicenter, randomized controlled trial examining the safety and efficacy of IM compared with IV midazolam in the prehospital setting is currently under way, and when completed in 2012 promises to better delineate the role of IM midazolam in prehospital seizure management.[36] Other potential areas of further research include airway management, alternative routes of medication administration, and the use of novel antiepileptic medications in the prehospital setting. Alternative routes of administration of medications frequently used in prehospital seizure management, such as intranasal or buccal midazolam, may be especially conducive to prehospital use, and warrant additional study. Antiepileptic medications that are not widespread in prehospital use such as propofol and fosphenytoin may also be worthy of study in the prehospital setting, particularly for seizures refractory to standard measures. Finally, the expanding evidence base on prehospital seizure management presents an opportunity for EMS medical directors to refine the prehospital seizure protocols in their EMS systems.

SUMMARY

Seizures are encountered frequently in the prehospital setting and are a leading cause of EMS activation and transport. EMS providers may encounter seizure patients when the seizure has prompted the 911 call, or when seizures occur in the setting of another chief complaint. The administration of benzodiazepines by paramedics directly affects patient outcomes in the ED. Although benzodiazepines are commonly recommended as the initial therapy for status epilepticus in the hospital setting, there are serious side effects to the medications that pose the risk of respiratory depression in the prehospital setting. Because most seizures terminate spontaneously, use of benzodiazepines by prehospital providers should be reserved for cases of status epilepticus. While diagnosing the specific cause of seizures during the prehospital phase of care is challenging, reversible causes such as hypoglycemia and hypoxemia must be identified and addressed. It is imperative that prehospital providers are trained to assess and stabilize patients with seizures.

KEY CONCEPTS

- Seizures are a leading cause of prehospital medical care, accounting for up to 8% of all EMS encounters.

- The prehospital management of seizure patients focuses on terminating the seizures, preventing their recurrence, identifying treatable causes such as hypoxia and hypoglycemia, and preventing further injury as a result of the seizure episode.

- Patients still convulsing on EMS arrival, and those who experience a recurrent seizure before returning back to their baseline mental status, should be considered to be in status epilepticus.

- Benzodiazepines are the treatment of choice for prehospital status epilepticus. While many prehospital protocols use intravenous diazepam, it is noted that midazolam is useful because it can be given IM, and that diazepam can be administered PR.

- Spinal precautions are not routinely indicated in uncomplicated seizure patients.

- After initial assessment by an ALS provider, patients with normal vital signs, a normal neurologic examination, and no significant comorbidities can be safely transported by basic life support providers.

- Refusal of care by prehospital seizure patients is a common occurrence. Patients wishing to refuse care should be informed of the high risk of recurrent seizure, and their decision-making capacity must be assessed.

REFERENCES

1. Johnston C, King WD. Pediatric prehospital care in a southern regional emergency medical service system. South Med J 1988;81(12):1473–6.
2. Joyce SM, Brown DE, Nelson EA. Epidemiology of pediatric EMS practice: a multistate analysis. Prehosp Disaster Med 1996;11(3):180–7.
3. Clawson J, National Association of EMS Physicians. Prehospital systems and medical oversight; chapter 17: emergency medical dispatch. 3rd edition. Dubuque (IA): Kendall/Hunt Pub; 2002.

4. Clawson J, National Association of EMS Physicians. Prehospital systems and medical oversight; chapter 18: priority dispatch response. 3rd edition. Dubuque (IA): Kendall/Hunt Pub; 2002.

5. Alldredge BK, Gelb AM, Isaacs SM, et al. A comparison of lorazepam, diazepam, and placebo for the treatment of out-of-hospital status epilepticus. N Engl J Med 2001;345(9):631–7.

6. Morimoto K, Fahnestock M, Racine RJ. Kindling and status epilepticus models of epilepsy: rewiring the brain. Prog Neurobiol 2004;73(1):1–60.

7. Donovan PJ, Cline DM, Whitley TW, et al. Prehospital care by EMTs and EMT-is in a rural setting: prolongation of scene times by ALS procedures. Ann Emerg Med 1989;18(5):495–500.

8. Martin-Gill C, Hostler D, Callaway CW, et al. Management of prehospital seizure patients by paramedics. Prehosp Emerg Care 2009;13(2):179–84.

9. McArthur CL 3rd, Rooke CT. Are spinal precautions necessary in all seizure patients? Am J Emerg Med 1995;13(5):512–3.

10. Adams J, Verdile V, Arnold R, et al. Patient refusal of care in the out-of-hospital setting. Acad Emerg Med 1996;3(10):948–51.

11. Stark G, Hedges JR, Neely K, et al. Patients who initially refuse prehospital evaluation and/or therapy. Am J Emerg Med 1990;8(6):509–11.

12. Drane JF. Competency to give an informed consent. a model for making clinical assessments. JAMA 1984;252(7):925–7.

13. Holroyd B, Shalit M, Kallsen G, et al. Prehospital patients refusing care. Ann Emerg Med 1988;17(9):957–63.

14. Mechem CC, Barger J, Shofer FS, et al. Short-term outcome of seizure patients who refuse transport after out-of-hospital evaluation. Acad Emerg Med 2001; 8(3):231–6.

15. Galustyan SG, Walsh-Kelly CM, Szewczuga D, et al. The short-term outcome of seizure management by prehospital personnel: a comparison of two protocols. Pediatr Emerg Care 2003;19(4):221–5.

16. Alldredge BK, Wall DB, Ferriero DM. Effect of prehospital treatment on the outcome of status epilepticus in children. Pediatr Neurol 1995;12(3):213–6.

17. Treiman DM. Pharmacokinetics and clinical use of benzodiazepines in the management of status epilepticus. Epilepsia 1989;30(Suppl 2):S4–10.

18. Rainbow J, Browne GJ, Lam LT. Controlling seizures in the prehospital setting: diazepam or midazolam? J Paediatr Child Health 2002;38(6):582–6.

19. Warden CR, Frederick C. Midazolam and diazepam for pediatric seizures in the prehospital setting. Prehosp Emerg Care 2006;10(4):463–7.

20. Chamberlain JM, Altieri MA, Futterman C, et al. A prospective, randomized study comparing intramuscular midazolam with intravenous diazepam for the treatment of seizures in children. Pediatr Emerg Care 1997;13(2):92–4.

21. Vilke GM, Sharieff GQ, Marino A, et al. Midazolam for the treatment of out-of-hospital pediatric seizures. Prehosp Emerg Care 2002;6(2):215–7.

22. Holsti M, Sill BL, Firth SD, et al. Prehospital intranasal midazolam for the treatment of pediatric seizures. Pediatr Emerg Care 2007;23(3):148–53.

23. Cereghino JJ, Cloyd JC, Kuzniecky RI, North American Diastat Study Group. Rectal diazepam gel for treatment of acute repetitive seizures in adults. Arch Neurol 2002;59(12):1915–20.

24. Fitzgerald BJ, Okos AJ, Miller JW. Treatment of out-of-hospital status epilepticus with diazepam rectal gel. Seizure 2003;12(1):52–5.

25. Kuisma M, Roine RO. Propofol in prehospital treatment of convulsive status epilepticus. Epilepsia 1995;36(12):1241–3.

26. Fischer JH, Patel TV, Fischer PA. Fosphenytoin: clinical pharmacokinetics and comparative advantages in the acute treatment of seizures. Clin Pharmacokinet 2003;42(1):33–58.
27. Sinha S, Naritoku DK. Intravenous valproate is well tolerated in unstable patients with status epilepticus. Neurology 2000;55(5):722–4.
28. Abarbanell NR. Prehospital seizure management: triage criteria for the advanced life support rescue team. Am J Emerg Med 1993;11(3):210–2.
29. Hoffman JR, Luo J, Schriger DL, et al. Does paramedic-base hospital contact result in beneficial deviations from standard prehospital protocols? West J Med 1990;153(3):283–7.
30. Shah MN, Bishop P, Lerner EB, et al. Derivation of emergency medical services dispatch codes associated with low-acuity patients. Prehosp Emerg Care 2003; 7(4):434–9.
31. Sporer KA, Youngblood GM, Rodriguez RM. The ability of emergency medical dispatch codes of medical complaints to predict ALS prehospital interventions. Prehosp Emerg Care 2007;11(2):192–8.
32. Michael GE, Sporer KA. Validation of low-acuity emergency medical services dispatch codes. Prehosp Emerg Care 2005;9(4):429–33.
33. Minambres GE, Antolinez EX, Infante CJ, et al. Generalized convulsive status epilepticus: analysis apropos of 57 cases. An Med Interna 2001; 18(6):294–7.
34. Shneker BF, Fountain NB. Assessment of acute morbidity and mortality in non-convulsive status epilepticus. Neurology 2003;61(8):1066–73.
35. Towne AR, Pellock JM, Ko D, et al. Determinants of mortality in status epilepticus. Epilepsia 1994;35(1):27–34.
36. University of Michigan. Paramedic treatment of prolonged seizures by intramuscular versus intravenous anticonvulsant medications (RAMPART). In: ClinicalTrials.gov [internet]. National library of medicine. Available at: http://clinicaltrials.gov/show/NCT00809146. Accessed July 30, 2010.

The Emergency Department Evaluation of the Adult Patient Who Presents with a First-Time Seizure

Andy Jagoda, MD*, Kanika Gupta, MD

KEYWORDS

• Seizures • Evaluation • Discharge • Diagnostic testing

The emergency physician faces many challenges in evaluating a patient after a seizure, as the differential diagnosis is broad and many conditions can mimic a seizure. A detailed history from the patient and witnesses is paramount, as well as a thorough physical examination focusing on vital signs and neurologic findings. Adult patients visiting the emergency department (ED) with first-time seizures fall into 2 groups. Patients in the first group include those with altered mental status, focal neurologic abnormalities, signs of infection or significant medical disorder that requires an extensive work-up. Patients in the second group, which is the focus of this article, are the adults who return to a normal baseline mental status after a first-time seizure. In the past, the extent of diagnostic testing required for the second group was controversial because most studies comprised diverse populations of varying ages and causes of the seizure (**Box 1**).[1–8]

In approximately 45% of patients with a first-time seizure no cause is identified, and less than 10% have a metabolic or toxicologic cause.[6–8] Other causes of first-time seizures include stroke, tumor, trauma, and infection, including human immunodeficiency virus (HIV). The history and physical examination provides the basis for risk stratifying patients with new-onset seizures and for formulating the diagnostic evaluation required in the ED.

DIAGNOSTIC TESTING
Laboratory Testing

Various studies have examined the usefulness of blood tests in evaluating a first-time seizure. The literature suggests the yield from laboratory tests is low, and their routine

Department of Emergency Medicine, Mount Sinai Hospital, Mount Sinai School of Medicine, 1 Gustave Levy Place, Box 1620, New York, NY 10029, USA
* Corresponding author.
E-mail address: andy.jagoda@mountsinai.org

Emerg Med Clin N Am 29 (2011) 41–49
doi:10.1016/j.emc.2010.08.004
0733-8627/11/$ – see front matter © 2011 Elsevier Inc. All rights reserved.

emed.theclinics.com

Box 1
Practice guidelines for management of unprovoked seizures in the emergency department (ED)

In an adult presenting with an apparently unprovoked first seizure, should an electroencephalogram (EEG) be ordered routinely?

> Recommendation 1 (level B): for an adult with an apparent unprovoked first seizure, the EEG should be considered as part of the neurodiagnostic evaluation, because it has a substantial yield

> Recommendation 2 (level B): for an adult with an apparent unprovoked first seizure, the EEG should be considered as part of the neurodiagnostic evaluation because it has value in determining risk of seizure recurrence

For an adult presenting with an apparent unprovoked first seizure, should a brain imaging study (computed tomography [CT], magnetic resonance imaging [MRI]) be ordered routinely?

> Recommendation 3 (level B): for an adult presenting with an apparent unprovoked first seizure, brain imaging studies using CT or MRI should be considered as part of the neurodiagnostic evaluation

For an adult presenting with an apparent unprovoked first seizure, should blood counts, blood glucose, and electrolyte panels be routinely ordered?

> Recommendation 4 (level B): there are insufficient data to support or refute routine recommendation of laboratory tests such as blood glucose, blood counts, and electrolyte panels for an adult presenting with an apparent unprovoked first seizure, although they may be helpful in specific clinical circumstances

For an adult presenting with an apparent unprovoked first seizure, should lumbar puncture be routinely performed?

> Recommendation 5 (level B): there are insufficient data to support or refute recommending routine lumbar puncture in the adult initially presenting with an apparent unprovoked first seizure; however, in special clinical circumstances (eg, febrile patients), it may be helpful

In an adult presenting with an apparent unprovoked first seizure, should toxicologic screening be routinely ordered?

> Recommendation 6 (level B): there are insufficient data to support or refute a routine recommendation for toxicology screening; however, it may be helpful in specific clinical circumstances

What laboratory tests are indicated in the otherwise healthy adult patient with a new-onset seizure who has returned to a baseline normal neurologic status?

> Recommendation 1 (level B): determine serum glucose and sodium levels on patients with a first-time seizure with no comorbidities who have returned to their baseline

> Recommendation 2 (level B): obtain a pregnancy test if a woman is of child-bearing age

> Recommendation 3 (level B): perform a lumbar puncture, after a head CT scan, either in the ED or after admission, on patients who are immunocompromised

Which new-onset seizure patients who have returned to a normal baseline require a head CT scan in the ED?

> Recommendation 4 (level B): when feasible, perform neuroimaging of the brain in the ED on patients with a first-time seizure

> Recommendation 5 (level B): deferred outpatient neuroimaging may be used when reliable follow-up is available

Which new-onset seizure patients who have returned to normal baseline need to be admitted to the hospital and/or started on an antiepileptic drug?

> Recommendation 6 (level C): patients with a normal neurologic examination can be discharged from the ED with outpatient follow-up

Recommendation 7 (level C): patients with a normal neurologic examination, no comorbidities, and no known structural brain disease do not need to be started on an antiepileptic drug in the ED

Data from American College of Emergency Physicians. Clinical policy: critical issues in the evaluation and management of adult patients presenting to the emergency department with seizures [systematic review]. Ann Emerg Med 2004;43:605–25.

use is not recommended. The history and physical examination will normally predict most metabolic disturbances, with glucose abnormalities and hyponatremia being the most commonly identified.[1,2,5,6] A retrospective chart review by Henneman and colleagues,[7] which excluded patients with trauma, drug ingestion, or diabetes, identified 333 adult patients with new-onset seizures in a 5-year period. Seven patients were found to have hyponatremia and 2 had hypocalcemia. However, it is unclear if the abnormalities were predicted or if they were the cause of the seizure. In a prospective study of 136 patients, Turnbull and colleagues[5] found 4 cases of hypoglycemia and 4 cases of hyperglycemia. Two of the cases of hypoglycemia were not suspected based on the history and physical examination. Tardy and colleagues[8] found 1 case in 247 patients of unsuspected hypoglycemia, and 4 cases of hyponatremia, of which only 1 was not suspected from the history. In a prospectively studied cohort of 98 patients with first-time seizure, Sempere and colleagues[6] found 1 case of unsuspected hyponatremia in a patient with psychogenic water ingestion. There are no prospective data to support extensive metabolic testing (eg, calcium, magnesium, phosphate) beyond a sodium and glucose determination in patients who are otherwise healthy and who have returned to baseline mentation. Patients with predisposing factors to metabolic derangements (eg, renal failure, malignancy, malnutrition, or those on diuretics) should, in general, receive a comprehensive metabolic evaluation, although there are inconclusive data to direct laboratory testing. Turnbull and colleagues[5] found 2 patients with hypocalcemia in a prospective study of 136 patients with new-onset seizure (1 with cancer and 1 with renal failure). Tardy and colleagues[8] reported 1 case of hypocalcemia but clinical correlation was not provided.

Based on a systematic review of the literature, the American College of Emergency Physicians' (ACEP) Clinical Policy on the initial approach to patients presenting with a chief complaint of new-onset seizure does not recommend extensive metabolic testing in patients who return to normal baseline.[9] This conclusion has also been reached in a practice parameter published by the American Academy of Neurology on the evaluation of first-time seizures in children.[10]

All women of reproductive age require a pregnancy test.[11] Pregnancy causes significant physiologic stress and can thus theoretically lower the seizure threshold in patients with an underlying focus. In 1 study of 59 patients with new-onset seizures in pregnancy, 14 patients were diagnosed with gestational epilepsy, a seizure disorder that occurs only during pregnancy.[11] Determination of pregnancy status may affect disposition, initiation of therapy, and management. Noneclamptic pregnant patients with new-onset seizures and no comorbidities, such as recreational drug use or HIV, still require a neuroimaging study and an electroencephalogram (EEG). If these tests are normal, it is reasonable to observe the patient without initiating pharmacologic therapy.

A drugs-of-abuse screen and alcohol level are considerations in patients with a first-time seizure, although there is no evidence that such testing changes outcome.[12–14] These tests are indicated when a patient has a seizure associated with a toxidrome or with altered mental status. However, a positive drugs-of-abuse screen does not necessarily prove causality for new-onset seizure and the patient still requires a neuroimaging study in the ED to direct management. Pesola and Westfal[14] reported 4 cases of cocaine-related seizures in 120 patients studied, although not all patients received the same tests and a direct correlation was not demonstrated. Seizure caused by alcohol intoxication or withdrawal is a diagnosis of exclusion, as alcoholics are at increased risk for electrolyte abnormalities and traumatic injuries.[15] Routine testing for drugs of abuse and alcohol is of unknown benefit, but may suggest a cause of new-onset seizures and help with future medical and psychiatric management.

Neuroimaging

The necessity and timing of neuroimaging for patients with new-onset seizure remain controversial for emergency physicians. Noncontrast head CT scans reveal abnormalities ranging from 3% to 40% in patients with first-time seizure, which includes two-thirds with focal lesions and one-third with diffuse cerebral atrophy.[7,8,16] The incidence of finding an abnormality is increased if the patient has a focal neurologic finding, focal onset of the seizure, history of malignancy, or HIV.[17] In 1 study of 247 patients with a first-time seizure, 117 CT scans were normal, and 130 were abnormal.[8] Of the abnormal CT scans, 85 showed focal lesions (eg, stroke or tumor), and 45 showed diffuse atrophy. Twenty percent of patients with a nonfocal examination and a first-time seizure had an abnormality identified on CT.[6,8]

Alcoholics, patients with head trauma, patients with HIV, and the elderly deserve special mention. A 1988 Denver study reported that of 259 alcohol-related new-onset seizures, 58% had abnormal head CT. A clinically significant lesion was present in 16 (6.2%), 7 of whom were alert and had nonfocal neurologic examinations and no history of trauma. Ten (3.9%) had a lesion that led to a change in clinical management.[18] This study emphasizes the importance of avoiding labeling alcoholics with a first-time seizure as having an alcohol-withdrawal seizure; it also emphasizes that alcohol is a comorbidity that drives the need for ED neuroimaging. Seizure related to mild traumatic brain injury is rare, but when it occurs it has been associated with a 47% increased incidence of intracranial bleeding.[19] Pesola and Westfal[14] reported that 6 of 26 HIV patients with a first-time seizure had an acute lesion found on CT, 2 of which were not otherwise suspected based on physical examination. The elderly are at risk for both stroke and malignancy, thus head emergent CT is required when presenting with a new-onset seizure in the ED.[8]

The question remains whether identifying the abnormality in patients with nonfocal neurologic examinations who are evaluated in the ED has an effect on patient outcome. This depends on the outcome measure used; identifying a lesion may direct disposition and argues in favor of neuroimaging in the ED. In 2007, the American Academy of Neurology updated previous guidelines on neuroimaging in patients with first-time seizure.[17] A multidisciplinary group with topic expertise conducted a literature review from 1966 to 2004. Based on the best available evidence the Task Force could only generate weak recommendations that included obtaining a CT in the ED in patients with a history or physical examination suggestive of a focal lesion, or a focal seizure with or without generalization: for all other patients, the Task Force concluded that acute neuroimaging is probably beneficial, but not mandatory and may be deferred if scanning is not immediately available.

Magnetic resonance imaging (MRI) is more sensitive than CT in detecting subtle alterations of brain structures and is often preferred by neurologists for evaluating first-time seizure. However, CT is better than MRI for detecting acute hemorrhage, which is a critical determination when evaluating new-onset seizure in the ED. In addition, CT is more widely and rapidly available in many EDs. There are currently no ED-based studies that have investigated the use of MRI. The joint practice guideline discussed earlier deferred recommendations on emergent MRI pending further study.

EEG is useful in determining the cause of seizure and quantifying recurrence risk. Emergent EEG recording is important in patients with persistent altered mental status and in those who may be difficult to diagnosis clinically, such as those in nonconvulsive status epilepticus (SE), pharmacologically induced coma, or in patients who have received a paralytic agent. Although EEG may be helpful and can facilitate antiepileptic drug (AED) treatment to terminate a seizure, no studies to date have shown that rapid EEG may improve outcome in patients with nonconvulsive SE. Access to EEG is limited in many EDs, and there are insufficient data to make definitive recommendations for its use in the acute setting. A practice parameter by the American Academy of Neurology reported that for adults presenting with a first seizure, a routine EEG revealed epileptiform abnormalities in approximately 23% of patients, and these were predictive of seizure recurrence. They recommend that EEG should be considered as part of the routine neurodiagnostic evaluation of adults presenting with an apparent unprovoked first seizure.[20]

Lumbar Puncture

A lumbar puncture (LP) is indicated in the work-up of first-time seizure in cases of suspected central nervous system (CNS) infection or suspected subarachnoid hemorrhage. In particular, patients with new-onset seizure who present with fever, severe headache, immunocompromised state, or persistently altered mental status should undergo an LP.[7,8,14,21] A retrospective cohort of 100 consecutive HIV-positive patients identified 14 cases of CNS infections on LP, however, clinical correlation was not provided.[22] In a prospective cohort, Sempere and colleagues[6] reported on 8 HIV-positive patients found to have a CNS infection as a cause of their seizure, 2 of whom were afebrile without meningeal signs.

A review of the literature found no cases of occult bacterial CNS infection manifesting as an isolated seizure, without fever or abnormal neurologic findings. An exception may occur in cases of partially treated meningitis. Although there are no adult studies, it has been reported that in the pediatric population, those who have been taking antibiotics and present with a complaint of seizure may have meningitis even if afebrile; LP should be seriously considered in these cases.[23] One retrospective study reported 4 cases of meningitis in seizure patients with normal physical examinations, but none had a bacterial cause. Most patients in this study did not receive an LP and indications for LP were not clear.[7]

HOSPITAL ADMISSION

The need for hospital admission is obvious in the critically ill patient. The dilemma arises when establishing disposition for the patient who has fully recovered without persistent neurologic symptoms in the setting of a first-time seizure. To determine which of these patients require hospitalization, it is necessary to identify a valid outcome measure that assesses the correctness of the decision. Useful measures would include seizure recurrence, morbidity, or mortality within a defined period.

The recurrence risk of unprovoked (eg, epileptic) seizures has been studied rigorously, but is generally reported in 1-year and 5-year recurrence rates.[24–28] These studies also generally excluded patients who had an identifiable cause of their seizure. The cause of the seizure and EEG findings are the best predictors of recurrence. Recurrence rates are lowest when no cause is identified and the EEG is normal.[26] Patients who have structural lesions on head CT or those with focal seizures that generalize secondarily have a 1-year recurrence risk of up to 65%. Those patients will most likely benefit from initiating AED therapy.[26]

Unfortunately, this information is not easily applicable in the ED setting where results of EEG and high-quality neuroimaging studies are often not available. In addition, the 1-year recurrence rate is not the most appropriate outcome measure from the standpoint of disposition from the ED. A more salient outcome is the short-term risk of recurrence, and in this respect, there is a paucity of data. One study compared adult patients presenting with first-ever seizures comprising multiple seizures within 24 hours versus first-time single seizure and it was found that those presenting with multiple seizures were no more likely to have seizure recurrence, irrespective of cause or treatment.[29] Only 1 study investigated the incidence of seizure recurrence within 24 hours of ED presentation.[8] This was a retrospective review of all adult patients admitted to the hospital with a first-time seizure during a 2-year period. The investigators reported a 19% seizure recurrence rate within 24 hours of ED presentation, decreasing to 9% if those patients with alcohol-related events or focal lesions on CT were excluded. However, the applicability of these results is limited because those patients with recurrent seizures were not well described, thus making it impossible to assess whether recurrence could have been predicted based on physical findings or comorbid factors. ED-based studies have reported rates of hospital admission, but the decision to admit was not standardized, and the ability of admission to improve outcomes was not studied.[8,30]

In summary, the most rational approach to admitting patients with first-time seizure should be based on the physician's risk assessment of the patient's overall condition, taking into account other symptoms, medical problems, and social factors, including the patient's access to follow-up care (**Fig. 1**). Patients with comorbidities including age more than 60 years, known cardiovascular disease, history of cancer, or history of being immunocompromised should be considered for hospital admission. At present, there is insufficient evidence to support a recommendation to admit or discharge the awake, alert, and stable patient who has returned to baseline mental status after a new-onset seizure.

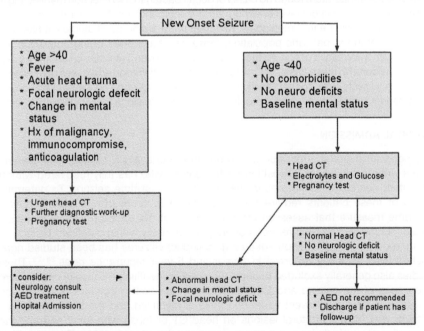

Fig. 1. Algorithmic approach to first time seizure. (*Data from* American College of Emergency Physicians. Clinical policy: critical issues in the evaluation and management of adult patients presenting to the emergency department with seizures [systematic review]. Ann Emerg Med 2004;43:605–25.)

INITIATION OF AED THERAPY

Preventing a seizure recurrence is the rationale behind starting an AED in the ED. Patients who have structural lesions on CT or patients with focal seizures that generalize secondarily have high risk (65%) of recurrence within 1 year, and are the group of patients that probably benefit from initiating AED therapy. However, identification of this subgroup requires laboratory testing, neuroimaging studies, and EEG, all of which are rarely immediately available in the ED. Moreover, AED treatment does not necessarily lower the risk of recurrence in all subsets of patients who have had a seizure. An uncontrolled study with a high rate of noncompliance reported a benefit for early initiation of AED treatment,[27] whereas an extended follow-up study of seizure recurrence by Hauser and colleagues[25] found that AED treatment was actually associated with an increased risk of recurrence. A study of patients with a history of traumatic brain injury has shown that phenytoin does not decrease the incidence of seizure recurrence.[31–33] There is no clear evidence-based data regarding initiation of AED treatment in adult ED patients with first-time seizures and this decision is best made in conjunction with the physician who will be providing long-term care for the patient.

SUMMARY

In the evaluation of a first seizure, determination of serum glucose and electrolytes is recommended, as is a pregnancy test in women of child-bearing age. A head CT should be obtained in the ED whenever feasible, but when reliable follow-up is available, it is acceptable to discharge the stable patient with no comorbidities for deferred outpatient evaluation. The decision to initiate anticonvulsant therapy is based on the patient's risk of recurrence, which is highest among patients with structural lesions on CT or focal seizure, which secondarily generalize. Because all AEDs have associated side effects, the risks and benefits of initiating pharmacologic therapy must be carefully weighed and discussed with the patient. Anticonvulsants are not recommended for patients with normal neurologic findings who lack comorbidities or known structural brain abnormalities. In this group, it is appropriate to withhold AED therapy pending the results of a complete diagnostic evaluation.

KEY CONCEPTS

- A serum glucose and electrolyte determination is indicated in adult patients with a first-time seizure who have no comorbidities and who have returned to their baseline. A pregnancy test should be obtained in women of child-bearing age.

- Ideally, neuroimaging of the brain in the ED should be obtained on all adults with a first-time seizure. If a head CT is not available in the ED, options include discussion of the risk of recurrence with the patient and with the patient's primary physician, and either admit the patient to the hospital or make arrangements for an outpatient evaluation versus deferred outpatient neuroimaging if reliable follow-up can be arranged.

- Patients with a first-time seizure do not require an LP unless they are immunocompromised, or have a fever, severe headache, or persistently altered mental status.

- Patients with a first-time seizure who have no known structural brain pathology, normal serum glucose and sodium levels, and a normal neurologic examination can be discharged from the ED with appropriate outpatient follow-up.

- Patients with a first-time seizure who have a normal neurologic examination and no known structural abnormality of the brain do not need to be started on an AED in the ED.

REFERENCES

1. Eisner RF, Turnbull TL, Howes DS, et al. Efficacy of a "standard" seizure workup in the emergency department. Ann Emerg Med 1986;15:33–9.
2. Powers RD. Serum chemistry abnormalities in adult patients with seizures. Ann Emerg Med 1985;14:416–20.
3. Kenney RD, Taylor JA. Absence of serum chemistry abnormalities in pediatric patients presenting with seizures. Pediatr Emerg Care 1992;8:65–6.
4. Rosenthal RH, Heim ML, Waeckerle J. First time major motor seizures in an emergency department. Ann Emerg Med 1980;9:242–5.
5. Turnbull TL, Vandenhoek TL, Howes DS, et al. Utility of laboratory studies in the emergency department patient with a new-onset seizure. Ann Emerg Med 1990;19:373–7.
6. Sempere AP, Villaverde FJ, Martinez-Menendez B, et al. First seizure in adults: a prospective study from the emergency department. Acta Neurol Scand 1992; 86:134–8.
7. Henneman PL, DeRoos F, Lewis RJ. Determining the need for admission in patients with new-onset seizures. Ann Emerg Med 1994;24:1108–14.
8. Tardy B, Lafond P, Convers P, et al. Adult first generalized seizure: etiology, biological tests, EEG, CT scan, in an ED. Am J Emerg Med 1995;13:1–5.
9. American College of Emergency Physicians. Clinical policy: critical issues in the evaluation and management of adult patients presenting to the emergency department with seizures. Ann Emerg Med 2004;43:605–25.
10. American Academy of Neurology. Practice parameter: evaluating a first nonfebrile seizure in children. Neurology 2000;55:616–23.
11. Knight AH, Rhind EG. Epilepsy and pregnancy: a study of 153 pregnancies in 59 patients. Epilepsia 1975;16:99–110.
12. Olson KR. Seizures associated with poisoning and drug overdose. Am J Emerg Med 1994;12:392–5.
13. Dhuna A, Pascual-Leone A, Langendorf F, et al. Epileptogenic properties of cocaine in humans. Neurotoxicology 1991;12:621–6.
14. Pesola GR, Westfal RE. New-onset generalized seizures in patients with AIDS presenting to an emergency department. Acad Emerg Med 1998;5:905–11.
15. Ng S, Hauser W, Brust J, et al. Alcohol consumption and withdrawal in new-onset seizures. N Engl J Med 1988;319:666–73.
16. Reinus WR, Wippold FJ, Erickson K. Seizure patient selection for emergency computed tomography. Ann Emerg Med 1993;22:1298–303.
17. Harden CL, Huff JS, Schwartz TH. Reassessment: neuroimaging in the emergency patient presenting with seizure (an evidence-based review): report of the Therapeutics and Technology Assessment Subcommittee of the American Academy of Neurology. Neurology 2007;69:1772–80.
18. Earnest MP, Feldman H, Marx J. Intracranial lesions shown by CT scans in 259 cases of first alcohol-related seizures. Neurology 1988;38:1561–5.
19. Lee ST, Lui TN. Early seizures after mild closed head injury. J Neurosurg 1992;76: 435–9.
20. Krumholz A, Wiebe S, Gronseth G, et al. Practice parameter: evaluating an apparent unprovoked first seizure in adults (an evidence-based review). Report of the Quality Standards Subcommittee of the American Academy of Neurology and the American Epilepsy Society. Neurology 2007;69:1996–2007.
21. Green SM, Rothrock SG, Clem KJ, et al. Can seizures be the sole manifestation of meningitis in febrile children? Pediatrics 1993;92:527–34.

22. Holtzman DM, Kaku DA, So YT. New-onset seizures associated with human immunodeficiency virus infection: causation and clinical features in 100 cases. Am J Med 1989;87:173–7.
23. Rosenberg NM. Seizures associated with meningitis. Pediatr Emerg Care 1992;8: 67–9.
24. Annegers JF, Shirts SB, Hauser WA, et al. Risk of recurrence after an initial unprovoked seizure. Epilepsia 1986;27:43–50.
25. Hauser WA, Rich SS, Annegers JF, et al. Seizure recurrence after a 1st unprovoked seizure: an extended follow-up. Neurology 1990;40:1163–70.
26. Berg AT, Shinnar S. The risk of seizure recurrence following a first unprovoked seizure: a quantitative review. Neurology 1991;41:965–72.
27. First Seizure Trial Group (FIR.S.T. Group). Randomized clinical trial on the efficacy of antiepileptic drugs in reducing the risk of relapse after a first unprovoked tonic-clonic seizure. Neurology 1993;43:478–83.
28. First Seizure Trial Group (FIR.S.T. Group). Treatment of the first tonic-clonic seizure does not affect long-term remission of epilepsy. Neurology 2006;67:2227–9.
29. Kho LK, Lawn ND, Dunne JW, et al. First seizure presentation: do multiple seizures within 24 hours predict recurrence? Neurology 2006;67(6):1047–9.
30. Krumholz A, Grufferman S, Orr ST, et al. Seizures and seizure care in an emergency department. Epilepsia 1989;30:175–81.
31. Temkin NR, Dikman SS, Wilensky AJ, et al. A randomized, double blind study of phenytoin for the prevention of post-traumatic seizures. N Engl J Med 1990;323: 497–502.
32. Hauser WA, Kurland LT. The epidemiology of epilepsy in Rochester, Minnesota, 1935 through 1967. Epilepsia 1975;16:1–66.
33. Centers for Disease Control and Prevention. Prevalence of epilepsy and health-related quality of life and disability among adults with epilepsy. South Carolina, 2003 and 2004. MMWR Morb Mortal Wkly Rep 2005;54:1080–2.

Generalized Convulsive Status Epilepticus in Adults and Children: Treatment Guidelines and Protocols

Peter Shearer, MD[a,b,]*, James Riviello, MD[c]

KEYWORDS

- Generalized convulsive status epilepticus • Benzodiazepines
- Refractory status epilepticus • Electroencephalography
- Status epilepticus • Non-convulsive status epilepticus

Generalized convulsive status epilepticus (GCSE) is a medical emergency associated with significant morbidity and mortality.[1] Like an acute myocardial infarction or stroke, the timing for intervention is critical, as prolonged seizure duration is associated with a greater number of complications and a higher likelihood of permanent neuronal damage. Although it is generally accepted that a benzodiazepine bolus and a phenytoin infusion are the preferred initial therapies for the management of seizures and GCSE, there remains a great deal of variability in the way in which GCSE is managed. Not only are there no nationally accepted specific GCSE treatment protocols, few medical centers have protocols that assure that status epilepticus (SE) is treated uniformly throughout the various care settings within the institution.

The 1993 publication in the *Journal of the American Medical Association* of the Epilepsy Foundation of America's Working Group on Status Epilepticus recommendations was one of the first coordinated attempts to provide guidance to clinicians who must terminate a prolonged seizure with minimal complications and morbidity.[2] Since that time, there have been numerous published SE treatment recommendations based on consensus opinion, case series, and local treatment preferences. There have also been published clinical trials that address which therapies are most effective

[a] Department of Emergency Medicine, Mount Sinai School of Medicine, New York, NY, USA
[b] Department of Emergency Medicine, University of Illinois College of Medicine, Chicago, IL, USA
[c] Baylor College of Medicine, Texas Children's Hospital, Houston, TX, USA
* Corresponding author. Department of Emergency Medicine, Mount Sinai School of Medicine, One Gustave L Levy Place, Box 1149, New York, NY 10029.
E-mail address: shearerp@nychhc.org

Emerg Med Clin N Am 29 (2011) 51–64
doi:10.1016/j.emc.2010.08.005
0733-8627/11/$ – see front matter © 2011 Published by Elsevier Inc.

emed.theclinics.com

at terminating SE. Most importantly, specific guidelines have been published that clarify the optimal sequence of medications to be delivered to a seizing SE patient, as well as the time course over which this should optimally occur.

DEFINING STATUS EPILEPTICUS

Over time, the definition of SE has changed as greater understanding of the disease state has occurred. At the most general level, SE constitutes prolonged seizure activity that overwhelms the body's compensatory mechanisms required to maintain homeostasis. The Epilepsy Foundation of America's Working Group on Status Epilepticus used the definition of SE as a seizure lasting 30 minutes or 2 or more seizures without full recovery of consciousness between episodes.[2] Lowenstein and colleagues[3] proposed an "operational definition" for treatment of GCSE in adults and older children (age >5 years): 5 minutes or more of either a continuous seizure or 2 or more discrete seizures between which there is incomplete recovery of consciousness. The Pre-Hospital Treatment of Status Epilepticus (PHTSE) study defined SE as seizure activity continuing longer than 5 minutes[4]; and the VA Cooperative Trial on Treatment of Generalized Convulsive Status Epilepticus used a definition of continuous seizure activity of greater than 10 minutes, or more than 2 seizures without full recovery of consciousness between seizures.[5]

GCSE can be the result of an acute event or a remote event (**Box 1**). The acute causes include metabolic abnormalities, infections, toxicities, vascular events, and acute traumatic brain injury. Remote symptomatic seizures are more likely related to past central nervous system (CNS) injuries such as prior head injury, anoxia, or stroke. Up to 50% of SE patients have no prior seizure history.

In general, the patients who are most often recognized in the emergency department (ED) to be in SE are those with GCSE. Although the majority of GCSE patients have seizures that are secondarily generalized, regarding the emergent evaluation and treatment of these patients, seizures and GCSE patients with primarily generalized SE are managed the same as those with secondarily generalized SE (see the article by Huff and Fountain elsewhere in this issue for further exploration of this topic.

Brain compensatory mechanisms may initially prevent neuronal injury from seizures, especially hypertension with increased cerebral blood flow. Lothman[6] outlined systemic and brain metabolism alterations that occur with prolonged GCSE: hypoxemia, hypercarbia, hypotension, and hyperthermia, with then a decreased brain oxygen tension, mismatch between the sustained increase in oxygen and glucose use and a decrease in cerebral blood flow, and depletion of brain glucose and oxygen. Treatment guidelines emphasizing what to do during the first 20 to 30 minutes assume that these compensatory mechanisms remain intact during incipient and early GCSE stages. However, brain compensation requires adequate airway, breathing, circulation, and cerebral blood flow, and there are situations in which compensatory mechanisms may be compromised. A de novo inpatient GCSE study had a higher morbidity and mortality, suggesting that those with an underlying illness are compromised and at a higher risk.[7]

INCIDENCE, MORBIDITY, AND MORTALITY

The incidence of GCSE among the general population ranges between 8 and 41 cases per 100,000,[1,8] with a GCSE mortality rate in adults of 10% to 40%.[9,10] In a California study, the overall rate of SE was 6.2 per 100,000, with higher rates in children younger than 5 years (7.5/100,000) and the elderly (22.3/100,000).[11] In children, GCSE is most common in the very young, especially in those younger than 2 years[12]; in this group,

| Box 1 |
| Causes of status epilepticus |

Infectious

  Meningitis

  Encephalitis

  Brain abscess

Vascular

  Ischemic stroke

  Subarachnoid hemorrhage

  Subdural hematoma

  Epidural hematoma

  Vasculitis

Metabolic

  Hyponatremia

  Hypoglycemia

  Hypocalcemia

  Hypomagnesemia

Toxic

  Cocaine, crack

  Tricyclics

  Anticholinergics

  Isoniazid

  Alcohol withdrawal

Tumors

Eclampsia

more than 80% have either a febrile or acute symptomatic (identifiable) etiology. In a population-based cohort of childhood epilepsy, 41 of 159 (27%) had GCSE. SE was more likely within the first 2 years after the epilepsy onset, and risk factors for status included remote symptomatic cause, age of onset 6 years or younger, and partial seizures.[13] The high morbidity and mortality seen in adult and pediatric SE patients is related to the direct neuronal injury associated with a prolonged seizure as well as the underlying cause of the GCSE, such as a space-occupying lesion or CNS infection. The 10-year mortality after a first episode of SE is 2.8 times greater than the general population.[14] The causes of SE differ in children from adults. The Richmond Study[15] included all ages from the same center; the most common cause of GCSE in adults was cerebrovascular disease (25.2%) whereas fever or infection (35.7%) was the most common cause in children. A recent medication change was a major factor in all ages: 20% in children and 19% in adults. Under 1 year of age there is more often an identifiable cause of GCSE, which can be treated along with the seizure, leading to a lower morbidity and mortality than GCSE after 1 year of age.[16] Idiopathic GCSE is rare during the first several months, and becomes more common after 6 months. Treatable causes for seizures in 31 infants younger than 6 months presenting to the ED included: 7% with infectious origins, one with pneumococcal meningitis; inborn errors of metabolism in 16%; electrolyte abnormalities in 16%, and trauma in 3%.[17]

Morbidity and mortality increase as the duration of the GCSE episode increases. For episodes that last longer than 60 minutes, the normal compensatory mechanisms that occur initially with seizures begin to fail, causing complications related to both cerebral hypoxia and direct neuronal death as well as systemic effects such as hypoxia, hypotension, hypoperfusion and metabolic acidosis, hyperthermia, rhabdomyolysis, and hypoglycemia.[18] The adverse outcomes associated with this decompensation include the development of cardiac dysrhythmias, pulmonary edema, ductal invasive carcinoma, and death.[19] Complicating the decompensation that occurs over time is the fact that the longer the seizure continues, the more difficult it is to terminate pharmacologically.[20,21] In one study, patients treated within 1 hour of continued seizure activity had an 80% likelihood of seizure termination versus a 40% to 50% likelihood of termination in patients for whom therapy was initiated after 2 or more hours.[19] Overall, the mortality of patients who seize for greater than 60 minutes approaches 30%.

INITIAL STABILIZATION

When managing SE patients who are actively seizing, the emergency physician must ensure adequate oxygenation and ventilation, secure intravenous access, initiate pharmacologic interventions, and plan to obtain diagnostic studies once the seizure episode has been terminated.

If the airway is secured using rapid sequence intubation, paralytic agents will stop the motor activity but not the abnormal neuronal firing associated with GCSE. Ongoing, uncontrolled, neuronal firing is associated with the release of excitatory amino acids and to calcium influx, which are associated with neuronal injury.[22,23] If prolonged paralysis is needed, electroencephalographic (EEG) monitoring is indicated to guide management.

Because hypoglycemia can frequently result in seizure activity, a bedside serum glucose determination is an essential first step. If the glucose level is less than 80 mg/dL, or if a rapid dextrose determination is unavailable and hypoglycemia is suspected clinically, 50 mL of 50% dextrose should be administered intravenously (IV) to adults, or 2 mL/kg of 25% dextrose to children. Thiamine, 100 mg is recommended with dextrose boluses in adult patients who appear malnourished or could have concomitant chronic alcohol abuse. If a CNS infection is suspected, empiric antibiotic therapy with ceftriaxone, 1 to 2 g IV and vancomycin, 1 g IV should be given pending head computed tomography (CT) and lumbar puncture. In children with fever and GCSE, the issue of meningitis is more complex: meningitis must be considered but a febrile seizure also may be the cause of GCSE, which would not indicate antibiotics (see article by Hampers and Spina elsewhere in this issue for further exploration of this topic). As with adults, prolonged seizure activity can cause an elevation in temperature. The decision to start empiric antibiotics in children should be made rapidly, related to the history, with a low threshold, to give the initial first dose of antibiotics for meningitis based on age and vaccination history.

DIAGNOSTIC TESTING
Laboratory Studies

When intravenous access is secured, serum electrolytes, calcium, magnesium, glucose, blood urea nitrogen (BUN), creatinine, and liver function testing should be performed, noting that hypomagnesemia should be suspected in seizing patients who are hypokalemic. If the patient is known to be taking an antiepileptic drug for which a laboratory assay is available, those levels should be sent. A serum toxicologic screen for ethanol, aspirin, acetaminophen, and tricyclic antidepressants should be considered as well as a urine sample for drugs of abuse, even though these toxins will most likely not influence the management of acute GCSE.

Lumbar Puncture

Although the collection of cerebrospinal fluid is essential when either CNS infection or subarachnoid hemorrhage is suspected, it is not mandated for all GCSE patients. It is noted that GCSE itself can induce fever and the presence of white blood cells in the cerebral spinal fluid (CSF pleocytosis), which could complicate making the diagnosis of CNS infections such as meningitis or encephalitis.[24,25] In general, when treating GCSE patients it is most important to begin empiric antibiotic or antiviral therapy, obtain neuroimaging, and defer the lumbar puncture until which time it can be done safely.

Neuroimaging

A noncontrast head CT scan should be considered for all GCSE patients once they have been stabilized. Although the use of paralytic agents may be considered to control the motor activity of the seizure and facilitate the CT scan, it is preferred to terminate the episode with the use of antiepileptic drugs, and when necessary use short-acting paralytic agents such as rocuronium to facilitate neuroimaging. There is no preferred role for magnetic resonance neuroimaging for the acute diagnosis and management of GCSE patients, given the logistical difficulties associated with this diagnostic modality.

Electroencephalographic Monitoring

Although EEG monitoring is not essential in the acute diagnosis and treatment of convulsive SE, its use should be considered when electrical (subtle) SE or generalized nonconvulsive SE are in the differential diagnosis. Subtle SE is a consideration whenever a GCSE patient remains comatose after the termination of the generalized seizure, whenever paralytics render the neurologic examination impossible, and whenever the patient is placed in a pharmacologically induced comatose state (see later discussion). This consideration is important in that up to 48% of patients in one series continued to have electrical seizures (subtle SE) on EEG monitoring during the 24-hour period after treatment for GCSE, despite having no clinical signs of ongoing convulsions.[26]

STATUS EPILEPTICUS TREATMENT PROTOCOLS AND GUIDELINES

There are numerous antiepileptic drugs that are available for use in the acute management of GCSE. Despite the publication of thousands of articles that address management, there are remarkably few randomized clinical trials that demonstrate superiority of one agent over another. The Epilepsy Foundation of America's Working Group on Status Epilepticus recommendations were, for the most part, consensus based. Attempts 10 years later to update these recommendations using evidence-based medicine methodology were hampered by the fact that there was only one published randomized clinical trial on the treatment of SE.[5] As such, there have been no updates of the Epilepsy Foundation of America Working Group's initial work.

Studies have shown that a GCSE treatment protocol proactively established can facilitate quality care when the medical emergency actually occurs.[27,28] However, in a survey of the UK Intensive Care Society, only 12% of hospitals used such a specific protocol.[29] In the United Kingdom, a 4-step guideline has been devised and implemented in 3 centers.[30] The protocol allows for an aggressive approach to GCSE with first line of therapy, followed by a refractory SE arm when needed. Such a protocol assumes that first-line therapy for GCSE will take at least 30 minutes to administer.

First-Line Therapies: Benzodiazepines and Phenytoins

The pharmacologic treatment of GCSE has changed in the past 20 years, with increasing evidence supporting the first-line use of benzodiazepines with less emphasis on phenobarbital. In addition, fosphenytoin and intravenous valproate have become available in the United States and are developing roles in many protocols.

Benzodiazepines

Intravenous benzodiazepines remain the first drugs of choice for SE. Both diazepam (0.2 mg/kg given at 5 mg/min) and lorazepam (0.1 mg/kg given at 2 mg/min) are equally effective in terminating seizures. Studies comparing the rates of termination of status in children between IV diazepam and lorazepam showed no difference.[31] Although diazepam has a longer half-life than lorazepam, lorazepam has a smaller volume of distribution, thus the CNS levels remain constant for a longer period of time.

A San Francisco study of out-of-hospital treatment of seizures compared the use of lorazepam, 2 mg intravenous push (IVP), repeated once if needed, diazepam, 5 mg IVP and repeated if needed, and placebo. Seizure activity terminated in 60% of the lorazepam-treated patients, 43% of diazepam-treated patients, and 21% of patients who received placebo.[4] The difference between lorazepam and diazepam in this study was not statistically significant. Complications such as hypotension, respiratory suppression, and arrhythmias were significantly less common with either benzodiazepine as compared with placebo. The study underlines the efficacy of benzodiazepine in terminating seizures and their safety in the prehospital setting.

A recent prospective, observational analysis of children with SE in the North London Convulsive Status Epilepticus in Childhood Surveillance Study (NLSTEPSS) found that not receiving prehospital treatment was associated with episodes that lasted for more than 60 minutes. The investigators also found that children who received more than 2 doses of benzodiazepines had GCSEs that lasted longer than 60 minutes and were associated with respiratory depression.[32]

When intravenous access is not available in a patient with SE, alternative routes of drug delivery must be considered. Both diazepam and lorazepam can be given rectally,[33] though intramuscular injection with midazolam is preferable. Midazolam is water soluble and rapidly absorbed from an intramuscular site.[34,35]

Phenytoin and fosphenytoin

Phenytoin is very effective in the termination of seizures, but its limitation is the rate at which it can be delivered. The dose is 20 mg/kg in a nonglucose solution, with a second dose of 10 mg/kg given if needed.[36] The infusion rate is limited to 50 mg/min (25 mg/min in the elderly and patients with cardiovascular disease), as hypotension may occur primarily due to the propylene glycol diluent. Phenytoin slows the recovery of voltage-activated sodium channels, thus decreasing repetitive action potentials in neurons. This effect on the myocardium can also lead to QT prolongation and arrhythmias. Although this is rare, cardiac monitoring is recommended during the infusion.[37] To maintain phenytoin solubility it is formulated at a pH of approximately 12, thus it is extremely toxic to the vascular walls and should be given through a large vein. Extravasation can be disastrous for the patient, resulting in extensive necrosis, namely the "purple glove syndrome."[38–40]

Fosphenytoin is a prodrug of phenytoin with an added phosphoryl group that makes it water soluble and allows a lower pH (the solution is buffered to pH 8.6–9).[41] Without the propylene glycol, fosphenytoin can be infused at rates faster than phenytoin, though hypotension can still rarely occur. The lower pH decreases vascular irritation and decreases tissue toxicity, allowing for intramuscular administration. The conversion half-life is 8 to 15 minutes.[42] For simplicity, fosphenytoin is measured in phenytoin equivalents (PE) and can be given at up to 150 mg PE/min. No controlled studies of the use of fosphenytoin in SE have been published.

Phenytoin cannot be given intramuscularly; fosphenytoin can, with rapid achievement of therapeutic serum drug levels within 1 hour (within 30 minutes in 40% of patients).[43] Of note, fosphenytoin is prepared as 500 PE/10 mL, that is, an intramuscular loading dose of 1000 PE would be a 20-mL injection. This volume can be safely given in the buttocks; however, many nursing protocols preclude use of this volume and defaults to physician administration.

The VA Cooperative Study compared 4 treatment arms for GCSE: diazepam (0.15 mg/kg) followed by phenytoin (18 mg/kg); lorazepam alone (0.1 mg/kg); phenytoin alone (18 mg/kg); and phenobarbital alone (15 mg/kg). The subjects were inpatients and were randomized to receive 1 of the 4 treatment arms. In the analysis they were divided into those with overt GCSE and subtle GCSE (those with coma and ictal activity on EEG with or without subtle motor activity.) There was no difference in effect of the 4 treatments when all subjects were compared, but analysis of the group with overt SE showed a significant difference in seizure control only between lorazepam and phenytoin alone.[13] Despite problems with the study design (the efficacy of drugs was assessed at 20 minutes before phenytoin could be fully infused for all patients), it is clear that lorazepam can control more seizures in 20 minutes than phenytoin alone, but that phenytoin in conjunction with diazepam (as it rapidly redistributes out of the CNS compartment) is equal to lorazepam alone for initial seizure management.

Other First-Line Therapies: Valproate and Phenobarbital

Valproate

Valproate has only recently become available in the United States in IV form.[44] Although experience with IV valproate and SE is limited to small studies in adults and pediatrics,[45,46] the potential advantage is its excellent safety profile. Although the recommended loading dose of 15 to 20 mg/kg in dextrose-containing solutions at a rate of 3 to 6 mg/kg/min, rapid bolus infusions have been safely administered.[47] In small studies on the use of IV valproate for GCSE it has been reported to terminate seizure activity in 42% to 80% of patients.[45] Further study is needed, but one would expect valproate to be useful in cases where benzodiazepine use is limited by hypotension and where there is a known hypersensitivity to phenytoin, or status resulting from noncompliance in patients on valproic acid.

Phenobarbital

Phenobarbital has often been advocated in the past as a first-line intervention for GCSE. It works on the γ-aminobutyric acid A ($GABA_A$) receptor, similar to the mechanism of benzodiazepines. One study demonstrated it to be equal to the combination of diazepam and phenytoin in the control of GCSE.[48] The VA Cooperative Study showed no difference between phenobarbital in controlling SE when compared with lorazepam or the combination of phenytoin plus diazepam.[5] The problem with phenobarbital is its potential to induce profound respiratory depression and hypotension from its vasodilatory and cardiodepressant effects. The respiratory depressant effects are compounded when used—as it typically is—after treatment with a benzodiazepine. It also has a long half-life, which can make complications difficult to manage.[13]

THERAPY FOR REFRACTORY STATUS EPILEPTICUS

If the initial therapies to control GCSE are not effective, it can be assumed that the patient is in refractory SE. It must be remembered that the first-line therapy with a benzodiazepine may modulate the motor signs of seizure activity so that it might appear that the seizure has terminated, whereas instead it may be persistent. All patients at this point should have their airway reassessed and intubation considered. Neurology consultation should be initiated to discuss the indications for emergent monitoring.

Current literature supports the use of continuous IV infusion of anesthetic doses of midazolam, a barbiturate, or propofol in the management of refractory SE. Inhalational anesthetics do not have a well-defined role and can be considered along with other potentially useful, but less well studied medications such as lidocaine, chloral hydrate, adenosine, and ketamine.[49–52]

Midazolam

Midazolam is often the preferred benzodiazepine for continuous infusion in the management of refractory SE because of its short duration of action and titratability. A loading dose of 0.2 mg/kg is followed by an infusion of 0.05 to 2.0 mg/kg/h.[53] Lorazepam can also be given as a continuous IV infusion; however, there are limited data on its use in status and its long half-life makes withdrawal more difficult. A recent systematic review of the literature reported that in 54 patients in refractory SE, intravenous midazolam, though effective in 80% of cases, was less effective than propofol or pentobarbital. Midazolam produced less hypotension than the other 2 medications.[54] In one small, retrospective study of IV midazolam and propofol, the mortality was 57% in the propofol group and 17% in the IV midazolam group, though the study had only 14 patients, was not randomized, and did not have the power to demonstrate significance in this difference.[55]

Propofol

Propofol is another $GABA_A$ agonist along with the benzodiazepines and barbiturates. There are limited studies of its efficacy in refractory SE, but there is evidence that it provides almost immediate suppression of seizure activity after a bolus infusion.[56] It is rapidly metabolized, and studies report rapid recovery from the propofol when the infusion is discontinued.

Propofol is dosed with a bolus of 3 to 5 mg/kg followed by a continuous infusion at 1 to 15 mg/kg/h. The limiting factor in its long-term and high-dose use is the propofol infusion syndrome of hypotension, lipidemia, and metabolic acidosis in both adults and children.[57,58] Propofol can cause nonseizure jerking movements and even induce seizures; EEG monitoring should be present.[59]

Anesthetic Barbiturates

Pentobarbital and thiopental are much shorter acting than phenobarbital. Thiopental is rapidly metabolized to pentobarbital. Both agents are highly lipid soluble and will accumulate in fat stores, leading to prolonged elimination. In a recent series of 12 intensive care unit patients in SE, high-dose thiopental terminated seizures in all of the patients.[60] However, one-third of the patients needed either dobutamine or norepinephrine to support their mean arterial pressure during therapy. The investigators also noted prolonged recovery time from the medication after the seizures had been suppressed. Thiopental has a less favorable side effect profile than pentobarbital. It is more lipid soluble and the metabolic pathway can become saturated, leading to an accumulation of thiopental and delays in recovery when stopped. For these reasons, pentobarbital is preferred when a barbiturate is used to manage refractory status.[10] Pentobarbital is loaded at 5 to 15 mg/kg over 1 hour. An infusion can be started at 0.5 to 10.0 mg/kg/h.[37]

CHOICE OF THERAPY FOR REFRACTORY STATUS EPILEPTICUS

There is very little empirical data to guide the choice of therapy in an evidence-based fashion. Treatment modality is often based on expert opinion and available resources (eg, IV midazolam may be preferred as it is more readily available in the ED than pentobarbital), and the patient's hemodynamic status.

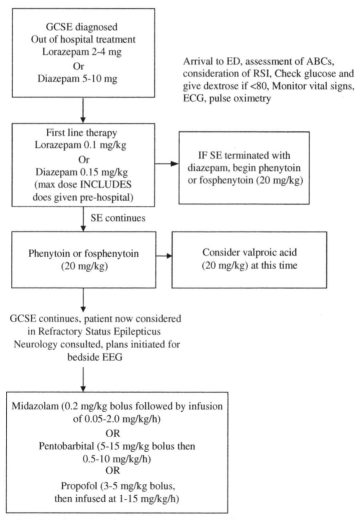

Fig. 1. Medication algorithm for the management of status epilepticus. ABCs, airway, breathing, circulation; ECG, electrocardiogram; ED, emergency department; EEG, electroencephalogram; GCSE, generalized convulsive status epilepticus; RSI, rapid sequence intubation; SE, status epilepticus.

A systematic review of the literature[37] did not find sufficient evidence to support the superiority of pentobarbital, propofol, or midazolam. Systematic reviews are only as strong as their respective data sources, and there is a lack of controlled studies in the treatment of refractory SE. Although the authors have found less treatment failure with pentobarbital or need to change to other medications compared with the other 2 drugs, there has also been more frequent hypotension with pentobarbital.

ALGORITHM FOR TREATING STATUS EPILEPTICUS

When a patient presents with GCSE, the time to termination of seizure may become dependent on the time it takes for the physician to choose a drug and for the nurse to administer it. Thus the ability of an ED to provide the rapid resources needed to treat SE depends on development of a prearranged treatment algorithm (**Fig. 1**). Preselection of medications for first-line use and those for refractory SE use will prevent delays when patients present. With a lack of strong evidence to select a preferred treatment for refractory SE, individual departments may make choices in conjunction with their neurology and critical care services, based on drug availability and on nursing familiarity with the given drugs.

Treatment in the prehospital arena begins with either IV lorazepam or diazepam. On presentation to the ED, continued seizure treatment begins with the stabilization of airway and vital functions. Initial medication choice is IV lorazepam (0.1 mg/kg) or diazepam (0.15 mg/kg), taking into account the dose of either medication given in the field. If diazepam terminates the seizure, it should be followed by phenytoin or fosphenytoin (20 mg/kg). If a benzodiazepines does not terminate seizure activity, phenytoin or fosphenytoin, 20 mg/kg should be administered. Intravenous valproic acid might be considered if the patient is known to have been controlled with valproic acid in the past.

If seizure activity continues, the patient is considered to be in refractory SE. Management choices include midazolam, propofol, and pentobarbital. As mentioned, the choice of medication for a given ED protocol is based on drug availability and prior planning with neurology and critical care.

SUMMARY

SE continues to have a high morbidity and mortality, despite the availability of numerous antiepileptic drugs that can be delivered parenterally in the acute setting. It has been demonstrated that GCSE patients are most effectively treated when a protocol is followed. As such, it would benefit all institutions to follow an SE protocol that specifies a diagnostic and treatment plan that takes place over the first 90 to 120 minutes of management. Clinical data and published guidelines and protocols support the initial use of a benzodiazepine followed by a phenytoin. These 2 therapies will effectively treat most SE patients within 60 minutes. In special cases there might be an indication for IV phenobarbital or valproate. Those that do not respond to these 2 initial therapies are considered to be in refractory SE, requiring the continuous infusion of midazolam, pentobarbital, or propofol. The diagnosis of subtle GCSE should be considered when a patient remains comatose, is paralyzed, or is being treated with a continuous-infusion antiepileptic drug: In these cases, an EEG should be performed as soon as is feasible in the ED or on disposition to the intensive care unit in order to maximize patient outcome.

KEY CONCEPTS

- The formal definition of SE using a 30-minute time frame is not an operational definition; seizure treatment should not be delayed more that 5 to 10 minutes.

- Early seizure management includes checking blood sugar, ensuring oxygenation, and suspecting infection or drug intoxication.

- First-line therapy for SE includes lorazepam IV (0.1 mg/kg) or diazepam (0.2 mg/kg); if diazepam is used, it should be immediately followed by a loading dose of phenytoin or fosphenytoin.

- Refractory SE is diagnosed after failure of first-line therapy and treatment should be protocol driven: Choice of medication is dependent on availability, ED capability, and hemodynamic status of the patient.

- Recommended treatments for refractory SE include: midazolam infusion (0.2 mg/kg bolus then 0.05–2.0 mg/kg/h); pentobarbital (3–15 mg/kg slow push [with hemodynamic monitoring] followed by infusion 0.5–10.0 mg/kg/h; or propofol 3–5 mg/kg bolus, infusion at 1–15 mg/kg/h).

- An EEG should be considered in patients who have been in convulsive SE to ensure that all seizure activity has ceased.

REFERENCES

1. DeLorenzo RJ, Hauser WA, Towne AR, et al. A prospective, population-based epidemiologic study of status epilepticus in Richmond, Virginia. Neurology 1996;46(4):1029–35.
2. Working Group on Status Epilepticus. Treatment of convulsive status epilepticus. Recommendations of the Epilepsy Foundation of America's Working Group on Status Epilepticus. JAMA 1993;270:854–9 [see comments].
3. Lowenstein DH, Bleck T, Macdonald RL. It's time to revise the definition of status epilepticus. Epilepsia 1999;40(1):120–2.
4. Alldredge BK, Gelb AM, Isaacs SM, et al. A comparison of lorazepam, diazepam, and placebo for the treatment of out-of-hospital status epilepticus. N Engl J Med 2001;345(9):631–7.
5. Treiman DM, Meyers PD, Walton NY, et al. A comparison of four treatments for generalized convulsive status epilepticus. Veterans Affairs Status Epilepticus Cooperative Study Group. N Engl J Med 1998;339(12):792–8.
6. Lothman E. The biochemical basis and pathophysiology of status epilepticus. Neurology 1990;40(5 Suppl 2):13–23.
7. Delanty N, French JA, Labar DR, et al. Status epilepticus arising de novo in hospitalized patients: an analysis of 41 patients. Seizure 2001;10(2):116–9.
8. Coeytaux A, Jallon P, Galobardes B, et al. Incidence of status epilepticus in French-speaking Switzerland: (EPISTAR). Neurology 2000;55(5):693–7.
9. Knake S, Rosenow F, Vescovi M, et al. Incidence of status epilepticus in adults in Germany: a prospective, population-based study. Epilepsia 2001;42(6):714–8.
10. Vignatelli L, Tonon C, D'Alessandro R. Incidence and short-term prognosis of status epilepticus in adults in Bologna, Italy. Epilepsia 2003;44(7):964–8.
11. Wu YW, Shek DW, Garcia PA, et al. Incidence and mortality of generalized convulsive status epilepticus in California. Neurology 2002;58(7):1070–6.
12. Shinnar S, Pellock JM, Moshe SL, et al. In whom does status epilepticus occur: age-related differences in children. Epilepsia 1997;38(8):907–14.
13. Sillanpaa M, Shinnar S. Status epilepticus in a population-based cohort with childhood-onset epilepsy in Finland. Ann Neurol 2002;52(3):303–10.

14. Logroscino G, Hesdorffer DC, Cascino GD, et al. Long-term mortality after a first episode of status epilepticus. Neurology 2002;58(4):537–41.
15. DeLorenzo RJ, Towne AR, Pellock JM, et al. Status epilepticus in children, adults, and the elderly. Epilepsia 1992;33(Suppl 4):S15–25.
16. Maytal J, Shinnar S, Moshe SL, et al. Low morbidity and mortality of status epilepticus in children. Pediatrics 1989;83(3):323–31.
17. Bui TT, Delgado CA, Simon HK. Infant seizures not so infantile: first-time seizures in children under six months of age presenting to the ED. Am J Emerg Med 2002; 20(6):518–20.
18. Lowenstein DH, Alldredge BK. Status epilepticus. N Engl J Med 1998;338(14): 970–6.
19. Jagoda A, Riggio S. Refractory status epilepticus in adults. Ann Emerg Med 1993;22(8):1337–48.
20. Walton NY, Treiman DM. Response of status epilepticus induced by lithium and pilocarpine to treatment with diazepam. Exp Neurol 1988;101(2): 267–75.
21. Lowenstein DH, Alldredge BK. Status epilepticus at an urban public hospital in the 1980s. Neurology 1993;43(3 Pt 1):483–8.
22. Meldrum BS, Vigouroux RA, Brierley JB. Systemic factors and epileptic brain damage. Prolonged seizures in paralyzed, artificially ventilated baboons. Arch Neurol 1973;29(2):82–7.
23. Which anticonvulsant for women with eclampsia? Evidence from the Collaborative Eclampsia Trial. Lancet 1995;345(8963):1455–63.
24. Aminoff MJ, Simon RP. Status epilepticus. Causes, clinical features and consequences in 98 patients. Am J Med 1980;69(5):657–66.
25. Quigg M, Shneker B, Domer P. Current practice in administration and clinical criteria of emergent EEG. J Clin Neurophysiol 2001;18(2):162–5.
26. DeLorenzo RJ, Waterhouse EJ, Towne AR, et al. Persistent nonconvulsive status epilepticus after the control of convulsive status epilepticus. Epilepsia 1998; 39(8):833–40.
27. Shepherd SM. Management of status epilepticus. Emerg Med Clin North Am 1994;12:941–61.
28. Appleton R, Choonara I, Martland T, et al. The treatment of convulsive status epilepticus in children. The Status Epilepticus Working Party, Members of the Status Epilepticus Working Party. Arch Dis Child 2000;83(5):415–9.
29. Walker MC, Smith SJ, Shorvon SD. The intensive care treatment of convulsive status epilepticus in the UK. Results of a national survey and recommendations. Anaesthesia 1995;50(2):130–5.
30. Garr RE, Appleton RE, Robson WJ, et al. Children presenting with convulsions (including status epilepticus) to a paediatric accident and emergency department: an audit of a treatment protocol. Dev Med Child Neurol 1999; 41(1):44–7.
31. Leppik IE, Derivan AT, Homan RW, et al. Double-blind study of lorazepam and diazepam in status epilepticus. JAMA 1983;249(11):1452–4.
32. Chin RFM, Neville BGR, Peckham C, et al. Treatment of community-onset, childhood convulsive status epilepticus: a prospective, population-based study. Lancet Neurol 2008;7:696–703.
33. Appleton R, Sweeney A, Choonara I, et al. Lorazepam versus diazepam in the acute treatment of epileptic seizures and status epilepticus. Dev Med Child Neurol 1995;37(8):682–8.

34. Chamberlain JM, Altieri MA, Futterman C, et al. A prospective, randomized study comparing intramuscular midazolam with intravenous diazepam for the treatment of seizures in children. Pediatr Emerg Care 1997;13(2):92–4.
35. Towne AR, DeLorenzo RJ. Use of intramuscular midazolam for status epilepticus. J Emerg Med 1999;17(2):323–8.
36. Browne TR. The pharmacokinetics of agents used to treat status epilepticus. Neurology 1990;40(5 Suppl 2):28–32.
37. Manno EM. New management strategies in the treatment of status epilepticus. Mayo Clin Proc 2003;78(4):508–18.
38. Kilarski DJ, Buchanan C, Von Behren L. Soft-tissue damage associated with intravenous phenytoin. N Engl J Med 1984;311(18):1186–7.
39. O'Brien TJ, Cascino GD, So EL, et al. Incidence and clinical consequence of the purple glove syndrome in patients receiving intravenous phenytoin. Neurology 1998;51(4):1034–9.
40. Burneo JG, Anandan JV, Barkley GL. A prospective study of the incidence of the purple glove syndrome. Epilepsia 2001;42(9):1156–9.
41. Rosenow F, Arzimanoglou A, Baulac M. Recent developments in treatment of status epilepticus: a review. Epileptic Disord 2002;4(Suppl 2):S41–51.
42. Browne TR, Kugler AR, Eldon MA. Pharmacology and pharmacokinetics of fosphenytoin. Neurology 1996;46(6 Suppl 1):S3–7.
43. Fischer JH, Patel TV, Fischer PA. Fosphenytoin: clinical pharmacokinetics and comparative advantages in the acute treatment of seizures. Clin Pharmacokinet 2003;42(1):33–58.
44. Devinsky O, Leppik I, Willmore LJ, et al. Safety of intravenous valproate. Ann Neurol 1995;38(4):670–4.
45. Giroud M, Gras D, Escousse A, et al. Use of injectable valproic acid in status epilepticus. Drug Investigation 1993;5(3):154–9.
46. Hovinga CA, Chicella MF, Rose DF, et al. Use of intravenous valproate in three pediatric patients with nonconvulsive or convulsive status epilepticus. Ann Pharmacother 1999;33(5):579–84.
47. Venkataraman V, Wheless JW. Safety of rapid intravenous infusion of valproate loading doses in epilepsy patients. Epilepsy Res 1999;35(2):147–53.
48. Shaner DM, McCurdy SA, Herring MO, et al. Treatment of status epilepticus: a prospective comparison of diazepam and phenytoin versus phenobarbital and optional phenytoin. Neurology 1988;38(2):202–7.
49. Walker IA, Slovis CM. Lidocaine in the treatment of status epilepticus. Acad Emerg Med 1997;4(9):918–22.
50. Pascual J, Sedano MJ, Polo JM, et al. Intravenous lidocaine for status epilepticus. Epilepsia 1988;29(5):584–9.
51. Lampl Y, Eshel Y, Gilad R, et al. Chloral hydrate in intractable status epilepticus. Ann Emerg Med 1990;19(6):674–6.
52. Yeoman P, Hutchinson A, Byrne A, et al. Etomidate infusions for the control of refractory status epilepticus. Intensive Care Med 1989;15(4):255–9.
53. Kumar A, Bleck TP. Intravenous midazolam for the treatment of refractory status epilepticus. Crit Care Med 1992;20(4):483–8.
54. Claassen J, Hirsch LJ, Emerson RG, et al. Treatment of refractory status epilepticus with pentobarbital, propofol, or midazolam: a systematic review. Epilepsia 2002;43(2):146–53.
55. Prasad A, Worrall BB, Bertram EH, et al. Propofol and midazolam in the treatment of refractory status epilepticus. Epilepsia 2001;42(3):380–6.

56. Brown LA, Levin GM. Role of propofol in refractory status epilepticus. Ann Pharmacother 1998;32(10):1053–9.
57. Cannon ML, Glazier SS, Bauman LA. Metabolic acidosis, rhabdomyolysis, and cardiovascular collapse after prolonged propofol infusion. J Neurosurg 2001; 95(6):1053–6.
58. Bray RJ. Propofol infusion syndrome in children. Paediatr Anaesth 1998;8(6): 491–9.
59. Makela JP, Iivanainen M, Pieninkeroinen IP, et al. Seizures associated with propofol anesthesia. Epilepsia 1993;34(5):832–5.
60. Parviainen I, Uusaro A, Kalviainen R, et al. High-dose thiopental in the treatment of refractory status epilepticus in intensive care unit. Neurology 2002;59(8): 1249–51.

Nonconvulsive Status Epilepticus

Andrew K. Chang, MD, MS[a],*, Shlomo Shinnar, MD, PhD[b]

KEYWORDS

- Nonconvulsive status epilepticus • Seizure
- Emergency medicine

Status epilepticus (SE) is a medical emergency, the morbidity and mortality of which can be decreased by prompt recognition and treatment. However, seizures can sometimes be of the nonconvulsive type and lack the dramatic convulsions that signal a typical tonic-clonic event. Without these overt motor manifestations, nonconvulsive seizures frequently go unrecognized, even by specialists, and can progress to nonconvulsive SE (NCSE).[1–3] Given the morbidity of SE in general, it is important for emergency physicians to recognize NCSE, although the time line to treat NCSE is controversial.[4,5]

NCSE is now known to be a heterogeneous disorder with varied causes and several subtypes. Despite evolving during the last 50 years, there is still no universally accepted definition. There is also disagreement on the electroencephalographic (EEG) features that are consistent with NCSE and confusion on how aggressively it should be treated, especially in patients who are critically ill and/or comatose.[6]

The 2 most commonly recognized types of NCSE are absence SE (ASE) and complex partial SE (CPSE). The primary clinical manifestation of both types of NCSE is altered mental status. It can be difficult differentiating these 2 types of NCSE based on clinical features alone,[7] and indeed there is little bearing on emergency management in making the distinction. The degree of mental status alteration can vary from mild confusion all the way to coma (**Box 1**). NCSE can either occur de novo or develop after a convulsive event, and it should be in the differential diagnosis of any patient with new-onset altered behavior of undetermined cause. When NCSE results in a coma, the condition must be differentiated from a convulsive seizure that has "burnt out," a condition termed subtle generalized convulsive SE or subtle SE (SSE).[8] NCSE and SSE should be suspected in patients who fail to wake up after a convulsive seizure and in those with coma of undetermined cause because they

The authors have nothing to disclose.

[a] Department of Emergency Medicine, Montefiore Medical Center, Albert Einstein College of Medicine, 111 East 210th Street, Bronx, NY 10467, USA

[b] Comprehensive Epilepsy Management Center, Montefiore Medical Center, Albert Einstein College of Medicine, 111 East 210th Street, Bronx, NY 10467, USA

* Corresponding author.

E-mail address: Achang3@yahoo.com

Box 1
Clinical manifestations of NCSE

Functional

  Slow mentation/responses

  Disorientation

  Confusion

  Psychosis

  Unresponsiveness

Motor

  Gross movements: positioning, raising, flexion or extension of extremities, head deviation

  Rhythmic myoclonias

  Twitches

Automatisms

  Mimicry

  Gestural

  Ambulatory

  Verbal

Data from Jagoda A. Nonconvulsive seizures. Emerg Med Clin North Am 1994;12(4):963–71.

---

may have had an unwitnessed seizure. SSE is generally associated with significant central nervous system (CNS) injury and unlike CPSE or ASE, carries a grave prognosis.[9]

EPIDEMIOLOGY AND ETIOLOGY

It is estimated that up to 25% of all cases of SE are of the nonconvulsive type.[10,11] In one study, it was reported that 58% of cases did not have a previous history of epilepsy.[12] In a prospective population-based study of SE, NCSE was documented in 14% of patients initially treated for CPSE with termination of the motor activity.[9] In a retrospective review of patients in the intensive care unit who were in coma of undermined cause, Towne and colleagues[13] reported that 8% (19/236) had NCSE.

Historically, ASE was considered more common than CPSE.[14] However, several recent investigations suggest that CPSE is underreported and more common than previously thought.[15–17] Because complex partial seizures may rapidly generalize, it is probable that many cases of CPSE have been mislabeled as ASE. De novo absence status has been reported in elderly patients with no prior history of epilepsy.[18–20] Until recently, it was thought that CPSE was equated with temporal lobe SE. However, it is now thought that CPSE is often related to extratemporal seizure origins[21] with a possible frontal lobe preponderance.[7,15,22] NCSE can result from focal processes, such as tumors and scars from past CNS events [23,24] or from global stimulants including electrolyte abnormalities,[25,26] drug toxicity,[27–30] alcohol consumption,[31] hyperthyroidism,[32] and benzodiazepine withdrawal.[10,18,33]

Epidemiologic data for SSE are limited. In a 10-year retrospective study, Lowenstein and Aminoff[34] identified 38 patients who met the criteria for SSE. Another prospective study found 19 cases during a 24-month period.[35] Based on animal studies, Treiman[36] hypothesized that SSE occurs by electromechanical disassociation that can evolve from inadequately treated convulsive SE, so that in spite of continuous EEG ictal discharges only subtle motor phenomena are generated. However, a clear evolution from convulsive status has been rarely demonstrated in humans.[34] Most cases have an associated severe underlying encephalopathy.[37]

CLINICAL PRESENTATIONS

The diagnosis of NCSE is often delayed because of its subtle presentations. In a retrospective review of 23 patients presenting to the emergency department with altered mental status, only 13 patients were diagnosed with NCSE in less than 24 hours.[38] The literature is replete with reports of patients presenting with altered mental status being initially misdiagnosed with a psychiatric disorder and only later diagnosed with NCSE, by either EEG or the onset of a motor seizure.[2,39,40] Fagan and Lee[1] described 8 patients who had NCSE manifesting as a postictal confusional state. The level of consciousness in their series varied from awake to comatose. Patients are also frequently misdiagnosed as having an amnestic syndrome, metabolic encephalopathy, or dementia. Patients with underlying medical conditions, such as mental retardation or dementia, may express nonconvulsive seizures in a manner difficult to recognize by the clinician who is unfamiliar with the patient. Often, the caregiver is the only one who can appreciate this qualitative difference from the patient's baseline status. Patients who have had stroke who seem clinically worse than what one would expect for the particular lesion involved or those who are recovering less rapidly than typical may also have concurrent NCSE; this concurrent presence of NCSE has been referred to as stroke plus by some investigators.[19]

The 3 major clues to the diagnosis of NCSE include an abrupt onset, fluctuating mental status, and subtle clinical signs such as eye fluttering and various automatisms. Automatisms represent involuntary, autonomic movements that occur with an alteration in consciousness, including those that are gestural (eg, picking movements with the fingers) or oroalimentary (eg, lip smacking).

Absence seizures (petit mal) are primarily generalized nonconvulsive seizures characterized by a sudden onset of unresponsiveness.[41] Simple associated automatisms, such as lip smacking, yawning, rubbing, or chewing, may accompany the seizure. The hallmark of ASE is a prolonged confusional state of variable duration and slowing of mental functions associated with a generalized EEG epileptiform alteration.[39,42] Although some patients may continue to function quite normally during ASE and only seem slightly less coordinated or alert,[5] the majority are lethargic, disoriented, and have decreased spontaneity and slow speech.[30]

Complex partial seizures, unlike simple partial seizures, are associated with impaired consciousness or disturbance of awareness. However, consciousness is usually not completely lost. Complex partial seizures usually begin with a cessation in verbal and motor activities associated with a motionless stare. Patients may be able to describe an aura before the event, which may help to distinguish a complex partial seizure from an absence seizure.

SSE occurs as a natural progression of untreated or insufficiently treated generalized tonic-clonic status epilepticus (GCSE) in which motor phenomena are exhausted.[6] Thus, convulsive motor activity is minimal but present, such as, eyelid, facial, or jaw twitchings; rhythmic nystagmoid eye jerks; or rhythmic subtle focal twitches of the trunk or extremities. These simple body movements are different from automatisms, which are refined patterned movements.[43] Despite these subtle movements, patients are stuporous or comatose and have bilateral EEG ictal discharges. **Table 1** compares and contrasts these various types of SE.

Table 1
Characteristics of NCSE and subtle generalized convulsive SE

	Absence	Complex Partial	Subtle Generalized
Typical clinical manifestations	Continuous or fluctuating confusion	Confusional state, usually with automatisms	Coma with subtle or no motor manifestations
EEG pattern	Generalized spike-and-wave pattern	Focal or secondarily generalized pattern	Generalized
Typical setting	History of seizures	History of seizures or focal brain lesion	Severe diffuse brain insult
Prognosis	Usually good	Usually good	Often poor

DIAGNOSTIC EVALUATION

The gold standard for diagnosing NCSE, including SSE, is an EEG.[44] **Box 2** lists some situations in which the diagnosis of NCSE (and hence an EEG) should be considered. Practically speaking, an EEG should be prioritized in patients with altered mental status for which no cause is identified. If such patients have a history of seizures, even if remote, the likelihood of NCSE is higher. NCSE should also be considered when the postictal state is prolonged, although the period that defines prolonged is variable and ranges from 30 minutes to 2 hours.[37,45] Other diagnostic tests are focused on identifying precipitants of NCSE, which include neuroimaging to evaluate for structural lesions, metabolic and toxicologic panels, pregnancy tests in women of childbearing age, and cerebrospinal fluid analysis in immunocompromised patients and those with fever and/or meningeal findings.

Obtaining an EEG may pose a significant dilemma for some systems where EEGs are not readily available,[44] and careful consideration must be given to the risk of delay in making a definitive diagnosis. Researchers have tried to develop predictive decision rules for selecting patients with an altered mental status for an EEG,[46] but as yet no model has acceptable sensitivity or specificity.

Empirical treatment with a benzodiazepine has been recommended to make the diagnosis of NCSE when an EEG is not immediately available. However, in general, it is preferred to obtain the diagnostic test before treatment because it will affect future decision making. In addition, patients with NCSE may not always respond readily to benzodiazepines. Thus, failure to improve does not exclude the diagnosis.

Box 2
Situations that should prompt consideration for the diagnosis of NCSE

1. Patients who have a generalized tonic-clonic seizure and a prolonged postictal period

2. Patients with altered sensorium, demonstrating subtle signs such as twitching or blinking and/or fluctuating mental status

3. Patients for whom no other cause is available to explain the altered sensorium, especially in those who have a history of a previous seizure, even if remote

4. Elderly patients with unexplained stupor or confusion, especially those taking neuroleptic medications

5. Stroke patients who look clinically worse than expected

TREATMENT

NCSE (not including SSE) has long been regarded as a benign entity because it does not produce the adverse systemic consequences of convulsive SE, such as hyperthermia, acidosis, hyperkalemia, pulmonary compromise, or cardiovascular collapse.[47] However, recent evidence suggests that the condition should be regarded as an emergency and should be treated quickly.[23,48–50] In general, the medications used to treat GCSE are also used to treat NCSE. Treatment should be given with simultaneous EEG monitoring to establish the therapeutic end point. Intravenous benzodiazepines are the first-line agents followed by intravenous phenytoin or fosphenytoin; conversely it is reasonable to use intravenous valproic acid as the second-line agent because theoretically it is more effective than the phenytoin in ASE.

The literature is unclear on the urgency of terminating NCSE in that no good functional performance studies are available correlating the duration of NCSE with outcome.[51] However, neuronal injury markers suggest cellular injury with NCSE,[23,52] and it is reasonable to aggressively treat the condition while addressing the underlying causes. Patients with SSE generally have significant underlying CNS injury with an associated high morbidity and mortality. Consequently, patients with SSE should be treated aggressively as any patient in refractory GCSE.

FUTURE DIRECTIONS

NCSE is a heterogeneous disorder. Work still needs to be done in developing a standardized definition and agreement on standardized terminology. Studies need to focus on the neuropsychological outcomes of the different subtypes of NCSE.[6] Finally, prospective multicenter studies are needed to determine the optimal treatment protocols for NCSE among different age groups and for different causes.

SUMMARY

NCSE, including subtle generalized convulsive SE, is primarily characterized by altered mental status. There should be a high index of suspicion in all patients with an altered mental status of unclear cause or with a prolonged postictal state. The diagnosis is made with an EEG. Treatment includes addressing underlying causes and aggressive pharmacologic interventions with a benzodiazepine, phenytoin, and valproic acid. The outcome is related to the underlying cause.

KEY CONCEPTS

- NCSE is a type of SE characterized primarily by altered mental status and should be suspected in patients with an altered mental status of unclear cause or with a prolonged postictal state.

- There are 2 main types of NCSE: the first is caused by a prolonged absence or complex partial seizure and the second, known as SSE, is the late manifestation of a prolonged generalized tonic-clonic seizure.

- NCSE is an underrecognized condition, especially in critically ill and comatose patients, and the delay in diagnosis and treatment may be associated with increased mortality (30% in SSE).

- The 3 major clues to the diagnosis of NCSE include an abrupt onset, fluctuating mental status, and subtle clinical signs such as eye fluttering, lip smacking, and picking movements with the fingers.

- NCSE should be managed initially with the administration of a benzodiazepine. SSE should be treated similar to generalized convulsive SE. The management of ASE and CPSE may vary to include an earlier use of intravenous valproate if a benzodiazepine fails to terminate the seizure activity.

REFERENCES

1. Fagan KJ, Lee SI. Prolonged confusion following convulsions due to generalized nonconvulsive status epilepticus. Neurology 1990;40(11):1689–94.
2. Guberman A, Cantu-Reyna G, Stuss D, et al. Nonconvulsive generalized status epilepticus: clinical features, neuropsychological testing, and long-term follow-up. Neurology 1986;36(10):1284–91.
3. Krumholz A. Epidemiology and evidence for morbidity of nonconvulsive status epilepticus. J Clin Neurophysiol 1999;16(4):314–22 [discussion: 353].
4. Thomas P. How urgent is the treatment of nonconvulsive status epilepticus? Epilepsia 2007;48(Suppl 8):44–5.
5. Cascino GD. Nonconvulsive status epilepticus in adults and children. Epilepsia 1993;34(Suppl 1):S21–8.
6. Maganti R, Gerber P, Drees C, et al. Nonconvulsive status epilepticus. Epilepsy Behav 2008;12(4):572–86.
7. Tomson T, Lindbom U, Nilsson BY. Nonconvulsive status epilepticus in adults: thirty-two consecutive patients from a general hospital population. Epilepsia 1992;33(5):829–35.
8. Treiman. Subtle generalized convulsive status epilepticus. Epilepsia 1984;25:653.
9. DeLorenzo RJ, Waterhouse EJ, Towne AR, et al. Persistent nonconvulsive status epilepticus after the control of convulsive status epilepticus. Epilepsia 1998; 39(8):833–40.
10. Dunne JW, Summers QA, Stewart-Wynne EG. Non-convulsive status epilepticus: a prospective study in an adult general hospital. Q J Med 1987; 62(238):117–26.
11. Celesia GG. Modern concepts of status epilepticus. JAMA 1976;235(15):1571–4.
12. DeLorenzo RJ, Hauser WA, Towne AR, et al. A prospective, population-based epidemiologic study of status epilepticus in Richmond, Virginia. Neurology 1996;46(4):1029–35.
13. Towne AR, Waterhouse EJ, Boggs JG, et al. Prevalence of nonconvulsive status epilepticus in comatose patients. Neurology 2000;54(2):340–5.
14. DeLorenzo RJ, Pellock JM, Towne AR, et al. Epidemiology of status epilepticus. J Clin Neurophysiol 1995;12(4):316–25.
15. Tomson T, Svanborg E, Wedlund JE. Nonconvulsive status epilepticus: high incidence of complex partial status. Epilepsia 1986;27(3):276–85.
16. Williamson PD, Spencer DD, Spencer SS, et al. Complex partial status epilepticus: a depth-electrode study. Ann Neurol 1985;18(6):647–54.
17. Cockerell OC, Walker MC, Sander JW, et al. Complex partial status epilepticus: a recurrent problem. J Neurol Neurosurg Psychiatry 1994;57(7):835–7.
18. Thomas P, Beaumanoir A, Genton P, et al. 'De novo' absence status of late onset: report of 11 cases. Neurology 1992;42(1):104–10.
19. Drislane FW. Presentation, evaluation, and treatment of nonconvulsive status epilepticus. Epilepsy Behav 2000;1(5):301–14.
20. Cascino GD. Complex partial seizures. Clinical features and differential diagnosis. Psychiatr Clin North Am 1992;15(2):373–82.
21. Lee SI. Nonconvulsive status epilepticus. Ictal confusion in later life. Arch Neurol 1985;42(8):778–81.
22. Williamson PD, Spencer DD, Spencer SS, et al. Complex partial seizures of frontal lobe origin. Ann Neurol 1985;18(4):497–504.
23. Krumholz A, Sung GY, Fisher RS, et al. Complex partial status epilepticus accompanied by serious morbidity and mortality. Neurology 1995;45(8):1499–504.

24. Varma NK, Lee SI. Nonconvulsive status epilepticus following electroconvulsive therapy. Neurology 1992;42(1):263–4.
25. DeLorenzo RJ, Towne AR, Pellock JM, et al. Status epilepticus in children, adults, and the elderly. Epilepsia 1992;33(Suppl 4):S15–25.
26. Kline CA, Esekogwu VI, Henderson SO, et al. Non-convulsive status epilepticus in a patient with hypocalcemia. J Emerg Med 1998;16(5):715–8.
27. Vollmer ME, Weiss H, Beanland C, et al. Prolonged confusion due to absence status following metrizamide myelography. Arch Neurol 1985;42(10):1005–8.
28. Ahmed I, Pepple R, Jones RP. Absence status epilepticus resulting from metrizamide and omnipaque myelography. Clin Electroencephalogr 1988;19(1): 37–42.
29. Callahan DJ, Noetzel MJ. Prolonged absence status epilepticus associated with carbamazepine therapy, increased intracranial pressure, and transient MRI abnormalities. Neurology 1992;42(11):2198–201.
30. Snead OC 3rd. Absence status epilepticus. In: Engel J Jr, editor. Epilepsy: a comprehensive textbook. Philadelpha: Lippincott-Raven Publishers; 1998. p. 701–7.
31. Fujiwara T, Watanabe M, Matsuda K, et al. Complex partial status epilepticus provoked by ingestion of alcohol: a case report. Epilepsia 1991;32(5):650–6.
32. Sundaram MB, Hill A, Lowry N. Thyroxine-induced petit mal status epilepticus. Neurology 1985;35(12):1792–3.
33. Thomas P, Lebrun C, Chatel M. De novo absence status epilepticus as a benzodiazepine withdrawal syndrome. Epilepsia 1993;34(2):355–8.
34. Lowenstein DH, Aminoff MJ. Clinical and EEG features of status epilepticus in comatose patients. Neurology 1992;42(1):100–4.
35. Altafullah I, Asaikar S, Torres F. Status epilepticus: clinical experience with two special devices for continuous cerebral monitoring. Acta Neurol Scand 1991; 84(5):374–81.
36. Treiman DM. Generalized convulsive status epilepticus in the adult. Epilepsia 1993;34(Suppl 1):S2–11.
37. Privitera MD, Strawsburg RH. Electroencephalographic monitoring in the emergency department. Emerg Med Clin North Am 1994;12(4):1089–100.
38. Kaplan PW. Nonconvulsive status epilepticus in the emergency room. Epilepsia 1996;37(7):643–50.
39. Andermann F, Robb JP. Absence status. A reappraisal following review of thirty-eight patients. Epilepsia 1972;13(1):177–87.
40. Berkovic SF, Bladin PF. Absence status in adults. Clin Exp Neurol 1983;19: 198–207.
41. Jagoda A. Nonconvulsive seizures. Emerg Med Clin North Am 1994;12(4):963–71.
42. Porter RJ, Penry JK. Petit mal status. Adv Neurol 1983;34:61–7.
43. Treatment of convulsive status epilepticus. Recommendations of the Epilepsy Foundation of America's Working Group on Status Epilepticus. JAMA 1993; 270(7):854–9.
44. Jordan KG, Schneider AL. Emergency ("stat") EEG in the era of nonconvulsive status epilepticus. Am J Electroneurodiagnostic Technol 2009;49(1):94–104.
45. Manno EM. New management strategies in the treatment of status epilepticus. Mayo Clin Proc 2003;78(4):508–18.
46. Husain AM, Horn GJ, Jacobson MP. Non-convulsive status epilepticus: usefulness of clinical features in selecting patients for urgent EEG. J Neurol Neurosurg Psychiatry 2003;74(2):189–91.
47. Manno EM, Pfeifer EA, Cascino GD, et al. Cardiac pathology in status epilepticus. Ann Neurol 2005;58(6):954–7.

48. Kaplan PW. The clinical features, diagnosis, and prognosis of nonconvulsive status epilepticus. Neurologist 2005;11(6):348–61.
49. Riggio S. Nonconvulsive status epilepticus: clinical features and diagnostic challenges. Psychiatr Clin North Am 2005;28(3):653–64, 662.
50. Riggio S. Psychiatric manifestations of nonconvulsive status epilepticus. Mt Sinai J Med 2006;73(7):960–6.
51. Drislane FW. Evidence against permanent neurologic damage from nonconvulsive status epilepticus. J Clin Neurophysiol 1999;16(4):323–31 [discussion: 353].
52. DeGiorgio CM, Gott PS, Rabinowicz AL, et al. Neuron-specific enolase, a marker of acute neuronal injury, is increased in complex partial status epilepticus. Epilepsia 1996;37(7):606–9.

Psychogenic Seizures: A Review and Description of Pitfalls in their Acute Diagnosis and Management in the Emergency Department

Matthew S. Siket, MD, MS, Roland C. Merchant, MD, MPH, ScD*

KEYWORDS

- Psychogenic seizures • Epileptic seizures
- Tonic-clonic seizures

The word seizure is derived from a Greek word, meaning "to take hold," and is popularly used to describe sudden and severe onset of symptoms.[1] When descriptively modified as epileptic, seizure is further defined as an event caused by abnormal electric discharges within the brain.[2] Nonepileptic seizures may resemble neurologic events but are not induced by neuronal hyperexcitation; instead, these seizures are classified as having either a physiologic or psychological cause. Physiologic causes include metabolic derangements, such as hypoglycemia and hyponatremia; organic brain lesions; cardiac arrhythmias; syncope; migraine headaches; and transient ischemic attacks. Psychogenic seizures (PS) originate from an underlying emotional trigger that may not be readily identifiable.

Reports of PS in the medical literature are long-standing. Hippocrates, a Greek physician, described hysterical epilepsy, and Aretaeus, a Greek physician, classified epilepsy into ordinary and hysterical.[3] Freud, an Austrian neurologist, further popularized the term hysteroepilepsy, which, along with simulated epilepsy and pseudoseizures, was used for many years to describe the same phenomena. Some prefer the term "psychogenic nonepileptic seizures" for this condition because it is thought to be less pejorative and more definitive than the previous diagnostic terms. The *International Classification of Diseases, Tenth Revision, Clinical Modification* labels PS as

Department of Emergency Medicine, Rhode Island Hospital, Alpert Medical School of Brown University, 593 Eddy Street, Claverick Building, Providence, RI 02903, USA
* Corresponding author.
E-mail address: rmerchant@lifespan.org

Emerg Med Clin N Am 29 (2011) 73–81
doi:10.1016/j.emc.2010.08.007
0733-8627/11/$ – see front matter © 2011 Elsevier Inc. All rights reserved.

dissociative convulsions, and the current *Diagnostic and Statistical Manual of Mental Disorders* (Fourth Edition, Text Revision) (*DSM-IV-TR*) describes this condition as a conversion disorder with seizures or convulsions, which implies that PS are most often unintentional.[4]

EPIDEMIOLOGY

The prevalence of PS among patients in the emergency department (ED) is unknown. It is estimated that the prevalence in the general population is between 2 and 33 per 100,000 persons.[5] Up to 30% of patients referred to epilepsy monitoring units are diagnosed with PS, and the mean delay between the onset of seizures and diagnosis of PS is 7.2 years.[6,7] An estimated $112,000 is spent on diagnostic evaluations and treatment of each patient with PS before the diagnosis is made.[8] Approximately one-third of patients with PS are treated for status epilepticus, and roughly one-quarter receive intensive care unit admission.[9] Most patients with PS are women aged between 20 and 30 years, although the diagnosis rarely has been made in patients older than 70 years.

ETIOLOGY

Most PS are considered to be a subtype of conversion disorders, wherein the physical symptoms are involuntary expressions of psychological distress. Although PS can occur in patients with factitious disorder and Munchausen syndrome and in those who are malingering, its occurrence is thought to be the exception rather than the rule.[10] More than 50% of patients with PS exhibit a history of other somatoform or dissociative disorders, and between 22% and 100% of patients fulfill the criteria for posttraumatic stress disorder.[4] In addition, several of the *DSM-IV-TR* Axis II personality disorders are associated with PS.[11]

Reuber[4] has suggested that in most patients, a combination of predisposing, precipitating, perpetuating, and triggering factors contribute to the development of PS. Multiple studies suggest that a history of sexual or physical abuse in childhood or adolescence is a major predisposing factor.[12] In addition, there seems to be a poorly understood genetic predisposition for PS.[13] Confounding the diagnosis of PS further is that between 5% and 40% of patients with PS have a concomitant diagnosis of epilepsy.[14] Although the relationship with epilepsy has been postulated by some to be largely because of modeled learning and observation, structural and functional brain abnormalities are found more commonly in patients with PS than the general population.[15] Among individuals potentially predisposed toward PS, precipitants such as major physical or emotional trauma, death of or separation from family members, job loss, legal action, and other significant life stressors have been linked to the development of this condition.[4] One study identified precipitating life events in all but 9% of patients with PS.[16] Suddenly occurring triggers have also been implicated in leading to PS in susceptible individuals, such as emergence from general anesthesia, sensory stimuli (eg, flashing lights, noises), and certain physical sensations. Patients with PS often become weary of emotional fluctuations, and it has been observed that these patients have greater fear sensitivity than healthy controls, which leads to isolation and avoidant behavior that further perpetuates the disease process.[17] Patients with PS are more likely than those with epilepsy to think that their health is determined by factors beyond their control, which explains why only half of the patients with PS engage in psychotherapy.[18–20]

DIAGNOSIS

The gold standard in the diagnosis of PS is prolonged video electroencephalographic (EEG) monitoring, a test which is not readily available in the ED. EEG alone is of limited utility unless direct observation is made of a typical episode of PS. Multiple studies have tried to identify clinical signs suggestive of PS, but none are individually sensitive or specific for the diagnosis.[21–23] Because no single feature is shared by all PS, it is important to consider all suggestive signs when considering the diagnosis.[24–26] Long duration, gradual onset, occurrence from apparent sleep, fluctuating course, asynchronous movements, pelvic thrusting, opisthotonus, side-to-side head or body movement, closed eyes during the episode, ictal crying, memory recall, absence of postictal confusion, and postictal stertorous breathing are all features that distinguish PS from epileptic seizures. The absence of intraoral lacerations and other forms of self-injury, urinary incontinence, impaired gag reflex, and extensor plantar response (Babinski reflex) also support the diagnosis but with very poor specificity. Vital signs can be helpful in supporting a diagnosis of PS when clinical suspicion exists. Ictal and postictal heart rates have been shown to be significantly higher in patients with convulsive epileptic seizures than in those with convulsive PS.[27]

Laboratory studies are of limited utility in the evaluation of a patient with suspected PS. After a generalized tonic-clonic seizure, a patient usually has some degree of lactic acidosis, as measured by a postictal lactate or blood gas analysis.[28] An elevated serum prolactin level has been shown to be highly predictive of generalized tonic-clonic and complex partial seizures but not in case of PS.[29] The elevation in serum prolactin levels is thought to be caused by a disruption in the hypothalamic regulation of pituitary hormone release after stimulation from temporal lobe epileptic foci.

It has been hypothesized that patients with PS have increased activity of neurobiological stress systems, manifesting as emotional hypervigilance, and can be measured using serum cortisol levels.[30] Although basal hypercortisolism may be present in some patients with PS, the level of cortisol has also been shown to be elevated after generalized and partial seizures, making it a poor differentiating diagnostic tool. A transient leukocytosis and elevated creatine kinase levels have also been observed after generalized seizures but not in PS, but neither is sensitive or specific enough to be of diagnostic value.[31,32]

Neuroimaging with magnetic resonance imaging (MRI) and single-photon emission computed tomography (SPECT) can be helpful in the diagnostic exclusion of PS. MRI can reveal a structural abnormality that may suggest an epileptic focus, but abnormal findings on MRI are also present in a large number of patients with PS.[15] Patients with PS most often have normal perfusion on SPECT, and a change in focal perfusion on an interictal SPECT compared with a postictal SPECT is highly suggestive of epilepsy.[33–35] However, the sensitivity and specificity of this imaging technique in PS are not well understood.

THERAPEUTIC MANEUVERS AND PROVOCATIVE TESTING

The use of sensory stimuli can aid in the diagnosis of PS and often results in termination of the event. Maneuvers such as placing a cotton swab in the nose, passively opening the patient's eyes, testing the corneal reflex, and the drop test are often met with resistance in a patient with PS but not in a patient with epileptic seizures. Eliciting a pain response with sternal rub or nail bed pressure and use of a noxious olfactory stimulus, such as anhydrous ammonia capsule under the patient's nose, may aid in the diagnosis and possibly terminate PS.[36] In addition, covering the patient's nostrils and mouth during an episode frequently causes the spontaneous termination of the episode and the return of spontaneous breathing.[37]

Geotropic eye movements have been shown to be highly suggestive of PS.[38] This test involves turning the patient's head from side to side while observing the patient's eyes. In patients with PS, voluntary saccades can be noted followed by deviation of the eyes away from the observer after the head is turned. Some patients with PS are highly suggestible and respond to verbal suggestions to both induce and terminate events.[24] Talking to patients during an episode, providing reassurance, and reminding them that they have the ability to control the seizure may be helpful in the diagnosis and management of PS.

The use of provocative testing to secure a diagnosis of PS is highly controversial.[39–41] These procedures are commonplace in tertiary epilepsy centers and are used to induce seizure activity in patients suspected of having PS. The most common procedure involves the injection of placebo (saline) that has been described to the patient as a proconvulsant agent, with an antidote (also placebo) available, if needed. Other techniques include photic stimulation and hyperventilation. Proponents of these techniques cite the gains of decreased cost, shorter time to diagnosis, and the avoidance of the adverse effects of prolonged use of antiepileptic drugs. Arguments against provocative testing cite ethical concerns of using deception and the irreparable damage it causes to the physician-patient relationship.

TREATMENT

Few studies have examined the effectiveness of therapeutic strategies in patients with PS.[9] Regardless, the first step is considered to be an open and nonconfrontational discussion explaining the diagnosis. Describing the seizure as functional, as opposed to psychogenic, might help in explaining the diagnosis to patients.[42] The use of antiepileptic drugs should be limited to those patients who have concomitant epilepsy. If a patient suspected of having PS is already receiving antiepileptic drugs, withdrawal of these medications should be restricted to the prescribing neurologist.

Behavioral therapy and operant conditioning have been proposed as potential psychological interventions for patients with PS. The primary goal of these techniques is to prevent rewarding of the seizures and to deliberately reward nonseizure activity in the hopes of extinguishing the episode of PS as a conditioned response to secondary gain.[14] Cognitive behavioral therapy has been shown to be effective in as few as 12 sessions of treatment.[43] Individual and group psychotherapy, hypnosis, and family therapy have also been described as methods of treatment of PS.[14,44,45]

Pharmacotherapy may be useful and should be directed at the underlying psychological disorder. Benzodiazepines can be effective in patients with underlying panic disorder and for patients who experience PS at night during sleep. Selective serotonin reuptake inhibitors have been suggested for other psychiatric comorbidities.[46]

PROGNOSIS

After receiving the initial diagnosis of PS, about 33% of patients become seizure free and 50% to 70% have a reduction in seizure frequency.[47] Prognosis seems to be highly dependent on and varies according to the type of underlying psychopathological condition. Approximately 25% of patients develop chronic PS, which has implications on driving restrictions, employment, and dependence on social security.[48]

PITFALLS IN THE ACUTE DIAGNOSIS AND MANAGEMENT OF PS

Although PS are among the most important diagnostic considerations for patients with seizures, this condition is not well understood and as a result, is often not well treated.[4] To secure a diagnosis of PS, a collaborative approach with a neurologist, preferably an epileptologist skilled in the use of video EEG monitoring equipment, and a psychiatrist is imperative. The ED is not an ideal environment to make this diagnosis, but failure to suspect the diagnosis can result in unnecessary administration of powerful sedatives, intensive care unit admission, endotracheal intubation, and the associated complications of these therapeutic measures, which include disability and death.[49] The following discussion highlights 4 ways in which the emergency medicine clinician can fall short in delivering optimal care to the patient with PS and provides some tips on how to avoid these errors.

Failing to Recognize the Signs of PS

In order to be diagnosed, PS must first be considered in the differential diagnosis. Because PS can resemble nearly any form of epileptic seizure, no single feature can be relied on as the sole trigger to raise a clinical suspicion of the presence of PS. It has been argued that historical components, such as the medical, social, and psychiatric history, are more helpful in differentiating PS from epilepsy than a description of the events themselves.[9] Several groups have tried to categorize the types of PS to assist in the ease of the diagnosis.[50–52] These categories have generally been divided into 2 types, those with predominant motor activity mimicking tonic-clonic seizures and those with a period of limpness, unresponsiveness, and/or altered mental status.[50] Another attempt at categorization separated PS into 3 types: swoons, often a nontraumatic fall followed by a period of limpness and eye closure without convulsion; tantrums with thrashing, convulsions, biting, and crying; and abreactive attacks characterized by initial overbreathing followed by stiffening, opisthotonus, breath holding or gasping, jerking, and pelvic thrusts.[51,52] Knowledge of common patterns of PS and vigilance for recognizing historical features suggestive of underlying psychopathological condition should help the emergency medicine clinician entertain the diagnosis when appropriate.

Inappropriate Diagnosis of PS

Because the emergency medicine clinician is challenged to make the diagnosis of PS without access to the gold standard test, mistakes are inevitable. A basic understanding of seizure symptoms and an awareness of uncommon manifestations of epileptic seizures are ways in which the clinician can prevent committing this type of error. These uncommon manifestations may mimic PS. For instance, bilateral arm movement with preserved consciousness can occur with myoclonic and temporal lobe epilepsy as well as when the epileptic foci involve the supplementary motor area of the brain.[53] Frontal lobe epilepsy can present with bizarre behavior if the supplementary motor area is involved or with strong emotions and fear if the cingulum (connecting the cortex to the limbic system) is affected.[9] Whenever there is clinical uncertainty as to whether a seizure pattern is neurogenic or psychogenic in origin, consulting a neurologist is advised.

Neglecting the Underlying Psychopathological Condition

The diagnosis of PS can be considered as a combination of a negative and positive diagnosis. The negative diagnosis is the determination that the seizures are nonepileptic. The positive diagnosis is the recognition of underlying psychological disease. The diagnosis of PS is therefore inappropriate if it has only been concluded that a patient's seizure is nonepileptic, without pursuing the underlying psychological cause that led to the event. This diagnosis is challenging in the ED, where patients are triaged by the perceived severity of their illnesses. After determining that a patient's seizures are nonepileptic and not life threatening, it may be difficult to take the time to address the underlying causative mechanisms. Completing this extra step, however, is necessary to appropriately care for the patient. This step is best achieved with an open and forthright discussion delivered in a nonjudgmental way that preserves patient dignity.[54] These conversations are often difficult, and many patients are initially angry. Whether the patients want to hear the diagnosis or not, it must be addressed to begin the process of relinquishing the sick role and transferring the responsibility from the health authorities to the patients themselves.[55]

Failing to Secure Adequate Follow-up

Whenever the diagnosis of PS is suspected, a collaborative team needs to be assembled to secure the diagnosis, including a neurologist, psychiatrist, and the patient's primary care physician. At the discretion of the consulting neurologist, certain patients should be referred to epilepsy monitoring units to have a video EEG performed to solidify the diagnosis. Outpatient treatment is often preferable to hospital admission.[52] Some patients may be resistant to seek follow-up and may engage in doctor shopping to validate their symptom complex.[6] Thus, securing follow-up with specific appointment dates and times is paramount.

FUTURE DIRECTIONS

Current research efforts are focused on the need to standardize treatment strategies for PS. Although cognitive behavioral therapy and psychotherapy have been established as effective treatment modalities, no randomized clinical trials have been published to date. LaFrance and colleagues[56] published results from a nationwide survey assessing the usual treatment of PS, in an effort to standardize treatment modalities, length of treatment, referrals, and cessation of antiepileptic medications. Further research is also being conducted on the use of a selective serotonin reuptake inhibitor in patients with PS.[46] Other research endeavors are aimed at using questionnaires in helping to distinguish PS from refractory epilepsy.[57] Patient- and family-centered assessment tools may be helpful in the diagnosis of PS in the acute care setting. Most studies of PS, including those analyzing the utility of provocative techniques, have been performed at epilepsy centers, so the utility of their data in the ED remains unclear.

SUMMARY

PS pose a challenge in the emergency medicine setting. The diagnostic gold standard is video EEG monitoring as interpreted by an experienced epileptologist, which is a tool unavailable to emergency medicine clinicians. The physicians must instead rely on their understanding of the clinical features, both historical and physical, that are suggestive of PS. When there is a clinical suspicion of this diagnosis, laboratory testing and therapeutic maneuvers can aid in differentiation from epileptic seizures. Assessment of underlying psychological distress is imperative, as is an open and honest discussion with the patient and family members about the diagnosis. After medical stabilization, the patient should be discharged with appropriate and timely neurologic and psychiatric follow-up. Recurrence is common, but with appropriate therapy, episodes can be significantly reduced, and complete resolution is possible.

KEY CONCEPTS

PS reflect an underlying psychiatric problem and do not have abnormal electric discharges on EEG. Patients with PS usually have a conversion disorder but might rarely have a factitious disorder or might be malingering.

Up to 30% of patients referred to epilepsy monitoring units for refractory seizures are diagnosed with PS. The mean delay between the onset of symptoms and diagnosis is more than 7 years.

No single clinical observation allows certain differentiation between PS and epileptic seizures, but long duration, gradual onset, occurrence from apparent sleep, fluctuating course, asynchronous movements, pelvic thrusting, opisthotonus, side-to-side head or body movement, closed eyes during the episode, ictal crying, memory recall, absence of postictal confusion, and postictal stertorous breathing are suggestive of a psychogenic cause.

Video EEG monitoring is considered the gold standard in diagnosing PS.

Treatment of PS involves addressing the underlying psychological stressor in combination with cognitive behavioral therapy or psychotherapy. Pharmacotherapy is of limited utility, and antiepileptic medication is ineffective.

Accurate diagnosis of PS is critical because it may avoid unnecessary testing or initiation of treatment with potentially harmful antiepileptic medications.

REFERENCES

1. Fisher RS, Boas WV, Blume W, et al. Epileptic seizures and epilepsy: definitions proposed by the International League Against Epilepsy (ILAE) and the International Bureau for Epilepsy (IBE). Epilepsia 2005;46(4):470–2.
2. LaFrance WC Jr. Psychogenic nonepileptic "seizures" or "attacks"? It's not just semantics: seizures. Neurology 2010;75(1):87–8.
3. Francis PA, Baker GA. Non-epileptic attack disorder (NEAD): a comprehensive review. Seizure 1999;8:53–61.
4. Reuber M. The etiology of psychogenic non-epileptic seizures: toward a biopsychosocial model. Neurol Clin 2009;27:909–24.
5. Benbadis SR, Hauser WA. An estimate of the prevalence of psychogenic nonepileptic seizures. Seizure 2000;9:280–1.
6. Friedman JH Jr, LaFrance WC. Psychogenic disorders. J Neurol 2010;67(6):753–5.
7. Reuber M, Fernández G, Bauer J, et al. Diagnostic delay in psychogenic nonepileptic seizures. Neurology 2002;58(3):493–5.
8. Souza D. Stereotypy of psychogenic nonepileptic seizures: insights from videoEEG monitoring. Methods 2010;51(7):1159–68.
9. Reuber M, Elger CE. Behavior psychogenic nonepileptic seizures: review and update. Science 2003;4:205–16.
10. Ozkara C, Dreifuss F. Differential diagnosis in pseudoepileptic seizures. Epilepsia 1993;34:294–8.
11. Bowman E, Markand O. Psychodynamics and psychiatric diagnoses of pseudoseizure subjects. Am J Psychiatry 1996;153(1):57–63.
12. Alper K, Devinsky O, Perrine K, et al. Nonepileptic seizure and childhood sexual and physical abuse. Neurology 1993;43:1950–3.
13. Kendler K, Aggen S, Czajkowski N, et al. The structure of genetic and environmental risk factors for DSM-IV personality disorders: a multivariate twin study. Arch Gen Psychiatry 2008;65(12):1438–46.

14. Bodde NM, Brooks JL, Baker GA, et al. Psychogenic non-epileptic seizures — definition, etiology, treatment and prognostic issues: a critical review. Seizure 2009;18:543–53.
15. Reuber M, Fernández G, Helmstaedter C, et al. Evidence of brain abnormality in patients with psychogenic nonepileptic seizures. Epilepsy Behav 2002;3(3): 249–54.
16. Bowman E, Markand O. The contribution of life events to pseudoseizure occurrence in adults. Bull Menninger Clin 1999;63(1):70–88.
17. Hixson J, Balcer L, Blosser G, et al. Fear sensitivity and the psychological profile of patients with psychogenic nonepileptic seizures. Epilepsy Behav 2006;9(4): 587–92.
18. Stone J, Binzer M, Sharpe M. Illness beliefs and locus of control: a comparison of patients with pseudoseizures and epilepsy. J Psychosom Res 2004;57(6): 541–7.
19. Golstein L, Drew C, Mellers J, et al. Dissociation, hypnotizability, coping styles and health locus of control: characteristics of pseudoseizure patients. Seizure 2000;9(5):314–22.
20. Howlett S, Grunewald R, Khan A, et al. Engagement in psychological treatment. Psychother Theor Res Pract Train 2007;44(3):354–60.
21. Walczak T, Bogolioubov A. Weeping during psychogenic nonepileptic seizures. Epilepsia 1996;37:208–10.
22. Chung S, Gerber P, Kirlin K. Ictal eye closure is a reliable indicator for psychogenic nonepileptic seizures. Neurology 2006;66:1730–1.
23. Vossler D, Haltiner A, Schepp S, et al. Ictal stuttering: a sign suggestive of psychogenic nonepileptic seizures. Neurology 2004;63:516–9.
24. Panagos PD, Merchant RC, Alunday RL. Psychogenic seizures: a focused clinical review for the emergency medicine practitioner. Postgrad Med 2010; 122(1):34–8.
25. Avbersek A, Sisodiya S. Does the primary literature provide support for clinical signs used to distinguish psychogenic nonepileptic seizures from epileptic seizures? J Neurol Neurosurg Psychiatry 2010;81(7):719–25.
26. An D, Wu X, Yan B, et al. Clinical features of psychogenic nonepileptic seizures: a study of 64 cases in southwest China. Epilepsy Behav 2010;17:408–11.
27. Opherk C, Hirsch LJ. Ictal heart rate differentiates epileptic from non-epileptic seizures [brief communications]. Neurology 2002;58(4):2001–3.
28. Lipka K, Bulow H. Lactic acidosis following convulsions. Acta Anaesthesiol Scand 2003;47(5):616–8.
29. Chen D, So Y, Fisher R. Use of serum prolactin in diagnosing epileptic seizures: report of the therapeutics and technology assessment subcommittee of the American Academy of Neurology. Neurology 2005;65(5):668–75.
30. Bakvis P, Spinhoven P, Roelofs K. Basal cortisol is positively correlated to threat vigilance in patients with psychogenic nonepileptic seizures. Epilepsy Behav 2009;16:558–60.
31. Shah AK, Shein N, Fuerst D, et al. Peripheral WBC count and serum prolactin level in various seizure types and nonepileptic events. Epilepsia 2001;42(11): 1472–5.
32. Holtkamp M, Othman J, Buchheim K, et al. Diagnosis of psychogenic nonepileptic status epilepticus in the emergency setting. Neurology 2006;66(11):1727–9.
33. Biraben A, Taussig D, Bernard A, et al. Video-EEG and ictal SPECT in three patients with both epileptic and non-epileptic seizures. Epileptic Disord 1999;1(1):51–5.

34. Varma A, Moriarty J, Costa D, et al. HMPAO SPECT in non-epileptic seizures: preliminary results. Acta Neurol Scand 1996;94(2):88–92.
35. Spanaki M, Spencer S, Corsi M, et al. The role of quantitative ictal SPECT analysis in the evaluation of nonepileptic seizures. J Neuroimaging 1999;9(4):210–6.
36. Lesser R. Psychogenic seizures. Psychosomantics 1986;27(12):823–9.
37. Massey E, Riley T. Pseudoseizures: recognition and treatment. Psychosomantics 1980;21(12):987–91; 996–7.
38. Rosenberg M. Geotropic eye movements and pseudoseizures. Arch Neurol 1986;43(6):544.
39. Benbadis SR. Provocative techniques should be used for the diagnosis of psychogenic nonepileptic seizures. Epilepsy Behav 2009;15:106–9.
40. Leeman BA. Provocative techniques should not be used for the diagnosis of psychogenic nonepileptic seizures. Epilepsy Behav 2009;15:110–4.
41. Kanner AM, Benbadis SR, Leeman B. Epilepsy & behavior rebuttals and a final commentary. Psychiatry (Abingdon) 2009;15:115–8.
42. LaFrance WC, Alper K, Babcock D, et al. Nonepileptic seizures treatment workshop summary. Epilepsy Behav 2006;8(3):451–61.
43. Golstein L, Deale A, Mitchell-O'-Malley A, et al. An evaluation of cognitive behavioral therapy as a treatment for dissociative seizures: a pilot study. Cogn Behav Neurol 2004;17(1):41–9.
44. Riggio S. Psychogenic seizures. Emerg Med Clin North Am 1994;12:1001–12.
45. Alsaadi T, Marquez A. Psychogenic nonepileptic seizures. Am Fam Physician 2005;72:849–56.
46. LaFrance W, Barry J. Update on treatments of psychological nonepileptic seizures. Epilepsy Behav 2005;7:364–74.
47. Iriarte J, Parra J, Urrestarazu E, et al. Controversies in the diagnosis and management of psychogenic pseudoseizures. Epilepsy Behav 2003;4:354–9.
48. Reuber M, House A. Treating patients with psychogenic non-epileptic seizures. Curr Opin Neurol 2002;15:207–11.
49. Morra VB, Coppola G, Orefice G, et al. Interferon-beta treatment decreases cholesterol plasma levels in multiple sclerosis patients. Neurology 2004;62:829–30.
50. Abubakr A, Kablinger A, Caldito G. Psychogenic seizures: clinical features and psychological analysis. Epilepsy Behav 2003;4:241–5.
51. Betts T, Boden S. Diagnosis, management and prognosis of a group of 128 patients with non-epileptic attack disorder, part I. Seizure 1992;1:19–26.
52. Betts T, Boden S. Diagnosis, management, and prognosis of a group of 128 correlates of intractable pseudoseizures. Part II, previous childhood sexual abuse in the aetiology of these disorders. Seizure 1992;1:27–32.
53. Rossetti AO, Kaplan W. Seizure semiology: an overview of the 'inverse problem'. Eur Neurol 2010;63:3–10.
54. Shen W, Bowman E, Markand O. Presenting the diagnosis of pseudoseizure. Neurology 1990;40:756.
55. Nordahl H, Loa B, Otto K. Changing the diagnosis from epilepsy to PNES: patients' experiences and understanding of their new diagnosis. Seizure 2010; 19:40–6.
56. LaFrance W, Rusch M, Machan J. What is "treatment as usual" for nonepileptic seizures. Epilepsy Behav 2008;12(3):388–94.
57. LaFrance WC, Devinsky O. The treatment of nonepileptic seizures: historical perspectives and future directions. Epilepsia 2004;45(Suppl 2):15–21.

Evaluation and Management of Pediatric Febrile Seizures in the Emergency Department

Louis C. Hampers, MD, MBA[a,b,*], Louis A. Spina, MD[c]

KEYWORDS

- Simple febrile seizure • Complex febrile seizure • Epilepsy

Pediatric febrile seizures are, by far, the most common form of first-time seizure in childhood. The incidence of a single febrile seizure is approximately 4% of all children younger than 5 years.[1] Because these occur in otherwise healthy children, an episode of generalized tonic–clonic convulsion represents an unfamiliar and terrifying event for most caregivers. These children are typically transported by emergency medical services (EMS) to the nearest emergency department (ED).[2,3] In fact, the caregivers' decision to activate the EMS system serves as a useful historical clue, particularly when the differential diagnosis includes febrile rigors. Very few parents will hesitate to dial 911 when witnessing a tonic–clonic seizure, and failure to do so may prompt the emergency clinician to consider nonconvulsive causes for the event.

CASE DEFINITIONS

For research and clinical purposes, pediatric febrile seizures have been divided into two categories: simple (typical) and complex (atypical).[4] The case definition of *simple febrile seizure* is rigid and exclusive. The definition of *complex febrile seizure* is less structured, essentially encompassing a heterogeneous group of pediatric seizures with fever that cannot be classified as simple febrile seizure.[4] To be termed a *simple febrile seizure*, a case must meet all of the criteria presented in **Box 1**. Strict application of this definition is important because this type of seizure has been extensively

[a] Section of Pediatric Emergency Medicine, University of Colorado School of Medicine, Denver, CO, USA
[b] Emergency Department, The Children's Hospital, Denver, CO, USA
[c] Division of Pediatric Emergency Medicine, Department of Emergency Medicine, Mount Sinai Medical Center, 1 Gustave L Levy Place, New York, NY 10029, USA
* Corresponding author. Section of Pediatric Emergency Medicine, University of Colorado School of Medicine, Denver, CO.
E-mail address: hampers.lou@tchden.org

Emerg Med Clin N Am 29 (2011) 83–93
doi:10.1016/j.emc.2010.08.008
0733-8627/11/$ – see front matter © 2011 Published by Elsevier Inc.

emed.theclinics.com

> **Box 1**
> **Clinical elements of simple febrile seizure**
>
> - Patient age between 6 months and 5 years
> - Generalized tonic–clonic convulsion
> - Spontaneous cessation of convulsion within 15 minutes
> - Return to alert mental status after convulsion
> - Documentation of fever (>38.0°C)
> - One convulsion within a 24-hour period
> - Absence of preexisting neurologic abnormality

studied and is known to have a benign prognosis.[4,5] Complex febrile seizures represent a heterogeneous population, and no literature supports a standardized approach to these cases. However, cases falling marginally outside the strict case definition of simple febrile seizures (eg, recurrent seizures, seizure of unclear duration, seizures associated with only tactile fever) most likely have a similarly benign prognosis. Patients far outside the definition (eg, a febrile 10-year-old in status epilepticus) must be carefully evaluated on a case-by-case basis.

CLINICAL ASSESSMENT

Patients who have experienced a febrile seizure will present more emergently than febrile age-matched "controls" without seizure.[2,3] Parental anxiety is typically high, and prehospital interventions such as intravenous line placement and supplemental oxygen can contribute to the child's distress. Perhaps because of the ominous implications of seizures accompanying fever in adults, clinicians historically have had a tendency to perform aggressive diagnostic workups on these children.[6]

If the case meets the definition of a *simple febrile seizure* (duration <15 min), the child unlikely will be convulsing on arrival to the ED.[7] In the immediate postictal state, the patient may be irritable, confused, lethargic, or even obtunded. Although rare, the phenomenon of a transient hemiparesis (Todd's paralysis) has been described in association with a simple febrile seizure; however, it suggests a focal origin and these cases warrant a careful evaluation.[8,9]

Most children with simple febrile seizure will gradually return to a normal level of alertness within an hour of the event. If the child does not appear toxic, distressed, or hemodynamically unstable, then a period of observation without further intervention is appropriate. If the child is capable of taking oral antipyretics, such as ibuprofen or acetaminophen, these should be administered, because the presence of fever may contribute to fussiness and make the clinical assessment more difficult. This observation period should be used to gather more historical information, which will be used to guide further management and discharge instructions. Key elements include the actual duration of the convulsion. EMS records of telephone activation and ambulance arrival are often useful when parents are unable to provide precise estimates. A history of seizures (febrile or afebrile) should be noted. A family history of epilepsy or febrile seizure is also contributory. A history of recent illness, and particularly documentation of fever, should be recorded.

LABORATORY TESTING IN PATIENTS WITH SIMPLE FEBRILE SEIZURES

Studies have shown that the measurement of serum electrolytes or glucose has no role in the evaluation of simple febrile seizures.[10–12] Similarly, no evidence suggests that emergent CT of the brain is useful in these cases.[11,13] The literature supports the finding that these children are at no greater risk for serious bacterial infection than age-matched controls who have not seized. In other words, the occurrence of a simple febrile seizure seems to contribute no independent risk for adverse outcome from infectious causes. In fact, the documentation of human herpes virus 6 as a causative agent in a large portion of febrile seizures implies that these children may actually have a lower risk of bacterial infection.[14,15]

Risk for Bacterial Meningitis

Because febrile seizure is common and bacterial meningitis by comparison is rare, no prospective study has directly assessed the relative risk of bacterial meningitis in this population. However, multiple retrospective studies have failed to show any increased incidence of bacterial meningitis associated with febrile seizure. Green and colleagues[16] retrospectively reviewed 486 pediatric cases of bacterial meningitis over a 20-year period, finding that 23% (111 patients) had experienced a seizure at presentation. Of those cases, only 7% (8 patients) were described as having a relatively normal level of consciousness. Of those patients, 6 presented with nuchal rigidity, 1 had experienced a prolonged focal seizure, and 1 had multiple seizures and a petechial rash. The authors concluded that all of the cases of bacterial meningitis that presented with seizure and a normal level of consciousness had an additional, clear indication for lumbar puncture.

Three other retrospective studies have looked at the incidence of bacterial meningitis in children presenting with febrile seizure.[15,16] Teach and Geil[15] reviewed 243 febrile seizures, of which 66 led to lumbar puncture. No cases of bacterial meningitis were found. Similarly, in a larger study, Trainor and colleagues,[17] reviewed 455 simple febrile seizures, of which 135 led to lumbar puncture. Again, no cases of bacterial meningitis were found. Most recently, Kimia and colleagues[18] reviewed 704 patients aged 6 to 18 months presenting with simple febrile seizures, 260 of whom underwent lumbar puncture. Once again, no cases of bacterial meningitis were found.

An obvious weakness of these reviews is that not all children presenting with febrile seizure were tested for bacterial meningitis. Nevertheless, if one presumes that the subset tested represented the youngest or most ill-appearing patients, the absence of bacterial meningitis among a total of 461 these cases suggests that the upper limit of the 95% confidence interval for the incidence of the disease in this "high risk" population is well below 2%. The literature is devoid of any description of a child who met criteria for simple febrile seizure with no other clinical indications for lumbar puncture who was subsequently found to have bacterial meningitis ("occult" bacterial meningitis).

The American Academy of Pediatrics published a practice parameter in 1996 regarding the approach to children with first-time febrile seizure.[4] Although acknowledging that the risk for bacterial meningitis was very low, and discouraging the "routine" performance of lumbar puncture, the guidelines urge clinicians to "strongly consider" this test in children younger than 12 months. The guidelines do not implicate febrile seizure as an independent risk factor, but rather assume that other clinical signs of meningitis may be more difficult to identify in this younger age group and that when uncertainty exists, clinicians should supplement their impressions with cerebrospinal fluid analysis.

Risk for Bacteremia

Similar to the risk for bacterial meningitis, the relatively low incidence of occult bacteremia presents a challenge for prospective work in this area. In addition, the success of the *Haemophilus influenza* vaccine has made some earlier studies less relevant to current practitioners.[19] Three retrospective studies have included patients in the post–*H influenza* vaccine era,[15,17,20] and all conclude that the likelihood of occult bacteremia is not affected by the occurrence of a febrile seizure.

In the studies by Teach and Geil[15] and Trainor and colleagues,[17] a subset of patients had blood cultures performed (206 of 243 and 315 of 455, respectively). Rates of occult bacteremia were low in both (2.9% and 1.3%, respectively). All pathogenic isolates were of *Streptococcus Pneumoniae*. In a similar retrospective cohort study, Shah and colleagues[20] examined the records of 379 children 2 months to 2 years old who presented with febrile seizure and had blood cultures performed. Occult bacteremia was noted in eight cases (2.1%), with all but one being *S pneumoniae* (one specimen contained Group A *Streptococcus*). The authors of all three studies concluded that the rates of bacteremia in children with febrile seizure were as low (or lower) as the "background" rate of bacteremia in febrile age-matched controls. Kimia and colleagues[18] did not directly address bacteremia in febrile seizures, and only discuss blood cultures in 10 patients found to have cerebrospinal fluid pleocytosis. However, none of these patients were found to have bacteremia.

The issue of appropriate investigations for occult bacteremia in all febrile toddlers is beyond the scope of this review, and has been the topic of extensive investigation and controversy. As pneumococcal vaccination further changes the probability and nature of this entity, the debate will continue.[21] However, the existing literature suggests practitioners should apply the same approach to patients experiencing a febrile seizure as that to the febrile toddler who has not had a seizure.[22]

Risk for Urinary Tract Infection

Little a priori evidence exists that children who have had a febrile seizure should have an increased risk for urinary tract infection (UTI). Two retrospective studies have reviewed the prevalence of UTI in these patients.[15,17] In Trainor and colleagues's[17] study, 171 children who had experienced a simple febrile seizure had urine cultures obtained. A total of 5.9% had cultures that grew more than 100,000 colony forming units of a pathogenic organism. This rate is similar to rates reported in prospective studies of other febrile toddlers, again leading to a conclusion that the occurrence of seizure does not alter the risk for serious bacterial infection. In their series, Teach and Geil[15] reported an even lower rate (0.7%) among the 130 patients cultured.

Risk for Bacterial Enteritis

The occurrence of seizures secondary to the presence of shigatoxin from *Shigella* enteritis has been well described.[23] Although the pathophysiology of these seizures differs from simple febrile seizure that is not toxin-mediated, the two entities may be clinically indistinguishable.[23,24] In the review by Trainor and colleagues,[17] 2 of 14 children who met criteria for simple febrile seizure were found to have *Shigella* enteritis, and all had a history of diarrhea. In the absence of additional data regarding the prevalence of *Shigella* in children meeting the case definition of simple febrile seizure, it seems sensible to culture those patients who have a history of bloody diarrhea or have recently traveled to an endemic area.

LABORATORY TESTS IN PATIENTS WITH COMPLEX FEBRILE SEIZURES

Complex febrile seizures include a heterogeneous array of conditions, and no standardized approach can be recommended. In each instance, the clinician must determine how far outside the definition of a simple febrile seizure a particular case falls.

Investigations should be directed at the elements that raise the greatest concern. For example, the febrile child in status epilepticus may be at risk for electrolyte abnormalities, toxic ingestions, traumatic brain injury, or meningitis. The febrile child who has had a brief, self-limited clinical seizure but remains obtunded should raise concerns for meningitis.[16,25] A child who has experienced a focal convulsion should raise the possibility of a brain abscess, mass lesion, or herpes encephalitis.[26]

Because of the heterogeneity of these cases, no literature quantifies a relationship between complex febrile seizure and the risk for serious bacterial illness. Regarding the risk of meningitis, the review conducted by Green and colleagues[16] may be instructive. Of 111 children with bacterial meningitis who had presented with convulsions, 103 were classified as *obtunded* or *comatose*, and the remainder all had some other clinical finding of concern (eg, nuchal rigidity), suggesting that seizure is a very late manifestation of central nervous system pathology in these infections.

Kimia and colleagues[27] also retrospectively reviewed the yield of lumbar puncture in 526 children presenting with a complex febrile seizure, among whom (64%) underwent a lumbar puncture. Of three patents diagnosed with acute bacterial meningitis, two grew *S pneumoniae* in the cerebral spinal fluid; one of these patients was described as being obtunded and the other had a bulging fontanel and apnea requiring intubation. The third patient was given a diagnosis of presumptive bacterial meningitis because of a positive blood culture for *S pneumoniae* with a negative cerebrospinal fluid culture. The cerebrospinal fluid was described as bloody and no sample was sent for cell count. Despite appearing well, the patient was treated empirically for bacterial meningitis with a 14-day course of antibiotics. These studies suggest that in an alert, otherwise well-appearing child, the occurrence of a febrile seizure with complex features per se cannot be considered a rigid indication for lumbar puncture.

Similarly, the decision to use empiric parenteral antibiotics (eg, ceftriaxone) should be based on the entire clinical picture, including other known risk factors for serious bacterial illness, such as toxic appearance, very young age, very high fever, and markedly elevated white blood cell count. For example, a 4-year-old who has had two convulsions within 24 hours but is well-appearing with an obvious viral stomatitis need not be considered at high risk for serious bacterial illness simply because a definition of complex febrile seizure has been met.

EMERGENT IMAGING IN PATIENTS WITH COMPLEX FEBRILE SEIZURES

The American Academy of Pediatrics practice guideline for the acute management of simple febrile seizures does not recommend emergency neuroimaging because intracranial abnormalities are rare in these patients.[4] No practice guidelines recommend emergent neuroimaging in patients presenting with a complex febrile seizure.

Teng and colleagues[28] performed a retrospective review of prospectively collected data examining the risk of emergent intracranial pathologic conditions in patients presenting with a first-time complex febrile seizure. During the study period, 79 patients presented with a first-time complex febrile seizure, 71 of whom were included in the analysis (2 were excluded for history of unprovoked seizure in the past, 4 for developmental delay, and 2 for lack of follow-up). From this group, 38 patients then underwent either CT or MRI (or both), although none were found to have an emergent intracranial pathologic condition.

Yucel and colleagues[29] performed a retrospective review of the neuroimaging results for 45 children presenting to the ED with a first-time complex febrile seizure. Although 7 (16%) patients were found to have abnormal CT or MRI findings, none required any emergent intervention. al-Qudah[30] also reported on the utility of neuroimaging in patients presenting with a febrile seizure, showing that none of 13 patients with complex febrile seizures had abnormal CT findings.

Garvey and colleagues[13] performed a retrospective review of neurologically normal children presenting to the ED with new-onset seizures (excluding simple febrile seizures) who underwent emergent neuroimaging. Of the 17 diagnosed with complex febrile seizures, 3 were found to have abnormalities on CT scan, none of which required emergent intervention.

These studies all suggest that emergent neuroimaging may not be necessary in well-appearing children presenting to the ED with a first complex febrile seizure.

As described later, although an indication for emergent neuroimaging may not be present, even well-appearing children who have had febrile seizures with complex features are at greater risk for epilepsy and will generally require subsequent evaluation with an EEG and neuroimaging studies. If these patients are to be discharged, an outpatient workup should be arranged.

DISCHARGE INSTRUCTIONS FOR CHILDREN WITH A SIMPLE FEBRILE SEIZURE

The prognosis for children who experienced a simple febrile seizure is excellent. However, most caregivers have just witnessed an extraordinarily stressful episode. Successful discharge instructions consist of information provided to parents in a clear, reassuring and understanding manner. In some cases an extended period of observation in the ED may be indicated simply to convince parents that a period of grave danger has passed.

Because by definition all cases have presented with a fever, patients always have at least 2 discharge diagnoses: one for the febrile seizure and a second for the cause of the fever. The source of the fever, if evident, should be managed in the standard fashion. Obviously, bacterial infections such as otitis media or sinusitis should be treated with antibiotics. For viral infections such as colds or gastroenteritis, instructions regarding the expected course of illness and home care recommendations should be provided. To address the caregivers' urgent concerns about the convulsion, these standard instructions must not be overlooked.

Risk of Recurrent Febrile Seizure

After a first-time febrile seizure, parents should be informed that the overall risk for a second febrile seizure before the sixth birthday is approximately 32%.[31] Although these recurrent seizures are also known to have a benign course, persuading caregivers that "home management" of subsequent convulsions is appropriate is difficult; clinicians must presume that the EMS system will again be activated. However, some management advice is appropriate. Clinicians should remind the parents to look at their watch or a clock at the onset of the seizure and ensure that the child is removed from an area with sharp or dangerous surfaces. Clinicians should explain that "swallowing of the tongue" is not a real concern, and discourage aggressive airway interventions such as bite-blocks.

The ED provider may use features of an individual case to more precisely quantify the risk of recurrence. In a prospective study of 428 children with first febrile seizure, Berg and colleagues[32] identified four risk factors associated with increased risk of recurrence, shown in **Box 2**. When no factors were present, the risk of a single recurrence was less than 15%. When all four factors were present, the rate exceeded 75%. Clearly, the caregivers of children with multiple risk factors should be informed of this high likelihood of recurrence.

Box 2
Clinical predictors of recurrent febrile seizure

- Patient younger than 18 months at first convulsion
- Temperature lower than 40.0°C at first convulsion
- Less than 1 hour between onset of febrile illness and first convulsion
- First-degree relative with history of febrile seizure

Prevention of Recurrent Febrile Seizure

Because fever is an obvious trigger for febrile seizure, it seems intuitive that antipyretics should have a role in lowering the incidence of recurrence. However, no literature supports this notion. In fact, several studies have failed to show that the prophylactic administration of acetaminophen or ibuprofen has any efficacy in this regard. In a prospective study of 104 children, Schnaiderman and colleagues[33] compared the use of round-the-clock acetaminophen at the onset of a febrile illness with sporadic doses for temperatures higher than 37.9°C. The recurrence rate in the study period was not significantly different between the groups (7.5% vs 9.8%, respectively). Similarly, van Stuijvenberg and colleagues[34] randomized 230 patients at high risk for recurrence to round-the-clock ibuprofen or placebo. The 2-year recurrence rates in the two cohorts did not differ significantly (32% vs 39%). Van Esch and colleagues[35] compared the recurrence rate of febrile seizure in 70 children randomized to round-the-clock acetaminophen or ibuprofen. Although the ibuprofen cohort had better fever control, no significant differences in the rates of recurrent febrile seizures were detected.

Most recently, Strengell and colleagues[36] performed a randomized controlled trial comparing the efficacy of different antipyretic agents for the prevention of febrile seizure recurrence. The study involved 231 children randomized into two groups: the first received rectal diclofenac and the second received rectal placebo. These groups were further randomized into three groups, with the children assigned to either oral ibuprofen, acetaminophen, or placebo. The patients were followed up for 2 years, with instructions to give the rectal medication at the onset of a febrile illness and begin the oral medication 8 hours later. This medication was given every 4 hours until the fevers resolved. The rates of febrile seizures between those who received placebo and those who received antipyretics were not significantly different (23.4% vs 23.5%; 95% CI, $-12.8–17.6$; $P = .99$).

The recommendation to administer round-the-clock antipyretics at the onset of subsequent febrile illnesses places a burden on caregivers. However, given the benign nature of recurrent febrile seizure and the lack of data supporting the role of antipyretics in reducing the recurrence risk, these strict instructions do not seem justified.[37] In fact, this advice may inadvertently contribute to "fever phobia" and make parents feel responsible for recurrences.[38–40]

For patients who have experienced multiple recurrences (more than three), referral to a pediatrician, neurologist, or pediatric neurologist may be appropriate. Although studies have shown efficacy in reducing the recurrence rate of febrile seizures using continuous antiepileptic therapy with phenobarbital, valproic acid, or primidone, and with intermittent oral diazepam,[41] this practice is not currently recommended.[5] Given the overall benign nature of a simple febrile seizure compared with the potential toxicities of antiepileptic therapy, the risks of treatment seem to outweigh the benefits. Rectal diazepam has been shown to give some benefit, and the American Academy of Pediatrics recommends the use of rectal diazepam when parental anxiety about febrile seizures is severe, because the medication may be effective in preventing recurrence.[42]

Risk of Epilepsy

Parents should be reassured that a self-limited generalized convulsion lasting less than 15 minutes is not associated with any long-term effects on brain function or intelligence.[43,44] However, they will often inquire about the risk of their child having, or developing, epilepsy. Using the most inclusive definition of epilepsy—more than a single afebrile seizure in a lifetime—caregivers can be informed that the risk of a child developing this condition after a single simple febrile seizure is very low. In the large British Birth Cohort study, the "background" rate of epilepsy was 0.4% by 10 years of age.[1] Children who had had a simple febrile seizure had a 1.0% risk. Although this represents a significantly increased relative risk, the overall prevalence remains low. To emphasize this, parents can be told that there is a 99% chance that their child will *not* have epilepsy.

Patients that do not meet the strict definition of simple febrile seizure (ie, recurrent, unprovoked seizures) have a much higher risk for developing epilepsy. The National Collaborative Perinatal Project identified three risk factors: family history of afebrile seizure, preexisting neurologic abnormality, and complex febrile seizure.[45] When all three factors were present, the risk for epilepsy was approximately 10%.

SUMMARY

Febrile seizure is a very common childhood condition. Although the recurrence rate is fairly high (roughly one-third), the overall prognosis is excellent and the risk of developing epilepsy is low (approximately 1%). The occurrence of a simple febrile seizure is not an independent risk factor for serious bacterial infection, and aggressive diagnostic evaluations are rarely indicated. Round-the-clock prophylactic administration of antipyretics have not been shown to affect the incidence of recurrence. Home administration of diazepam should be reserved for cases of multiple recurrences, and is best managed by a physician who will maintain a long-term, longitudinal relationship with the child's family.

KEY CONCEPTS

- The diagnostic workup for a child with a simple febrile seizure is the same as that for an age-matched febrile patient who did not have a seizure; these children are not at higher risk for bacteremia.

- Measuring serum electrolytes and spinal fluid analysis have no role in managing patients older than 12 months with simple febrile seizure; a lumbar puncture should be considered in patients younger than 12 months.

- Complex febrile seizures suggest the possibility of a significant underlying central nervous system pathology and these patients require a comprehensive evaluation.

- Patients with a simple febrile seizure have a 30% incidence of recurrence before their sixth birthday; subsequent use of antipyretics at fever onset does not lower the recurrence rate.

- Patients who have had a simple febrile seizure have a 1% lifetime risk of developing epilepsy versus a 0.4% risk in the general population.

REFERENCES

1. Verity CM, Golding J. Risk of epilepsy after febrile convulsions: a national cohort study. BMJ 1991;303:1373–6.
2. Smith RA, Martland T, Lowry MF. Children with seizures presenting to accident and emergency. J Accid Emerg Med 1996;13:54–8.
3. Johnston C, King WD. Pediatric prehospital care in a southern regional emergency medical service system. South Med J 1988;81:1473–6.
4. Practice parameter: the neurodiagnostic evaluation of the child with a first simple febrile seizure. American Academy of Pediatrics. Provisional Committee on Quality Improvement, Subcommittee on Febrile Seizures. Pediatrics 1996;97:769–72.
5. Duffner PK, Baumann RJ, Green JL, et al. Febrile seizures: clinical practice guideline for the long-term management of the child with simple febrile seizures. American Academy of Pediatrics. Steering Committee on Quality Improvement and Management. Subcommittee of Febrile Seizures. Pediatrics 2008;121:1281–6.
6. Hampers LC, Trainor JL, Listernick R, et al. Setting based practice variation in the management of simple febrile seizure. Acad Emerg Med 2000;7:21–7.
7. Knudsen FU. Febrile seizures: treatment and prognosis. Epilepsia 2000;41:2–9.
8. Rolak LA, Rutecki P, Ashizawa T, et al. Clinical features of Todd's post-epileptic paralysis. J Neurol Neurosurg Psychiatry 1992;55:63–4.
9. Leutmezer F, Baumgartner C. Postictal signs of lateralizing and localizing significance. Epileptic Disord 2002;4:43–8.
10. Rutter N, Smales OR. Calcium, magnesium, and glucose levels in blood and CSF of children with febrile convulsions. Arch Dis Child 1976;51:141–3.
11. Gerber MA, Berliner BC. The child with a "simple" febrile seizure. Appropriate diagnostic evaluation. Am J Dis Child 1981;135:431–3.
12. Jaffe M, Bar-Joseph G, Tirosh E. Fever and convulsions—indications for laboratory investigations. Pediatrics. 1981;57:729–31.
13. Garvey MA, Gaillard WD, Rusin JA, et al. Emergency brain computed tomography in children with seizures: who is most likely to benefit? J Pediatr 1998;133:664–9.
14. Barone SR, Kaplan MH, Krilov LR. Human herpesvirus-6 infection in children with first febrile seizures. J Pediatr 1995;127:95–7.
15. Teach S, Geil P. Incidence of bacteremia, urinary tract infections and unsuspected bacterial meningitis in children with febrile seizures. Pediatr Emerg Care 1999;15:9–12.
16. Green SM, Rothrock SG, Clem KJ, et al. Can seizures be the sole manifestation of meningitis in febrile children? Pediatrics 1993;92:527–34.
17. Trainor JL, Hampers LC, Krug SE, et al. Children with first-time simple febrile seizures are at low risk of serious bacterial illness. Acad Emerg Med 2001;8:781–7.
18. Kimia AA, Capraro AJ, Harper MD, et al. Utility of lumbar puncture for first febrile seizure among children 6 months to 18 months of age. Pediatrics 2009;123:6–12.
19. Chamberlin JM, Gorman RL. Occult bacteremia in children with simple febrile seizures. Am J Dis Child 1988;142:1073–6.
20. Shah SS, Alpern ER, Zwerling L, et al. Low risk of bacteremia in children with febrile seizures. Arch Pediatr Adolesc Med 2002;156:469–72.
21. Baraff LJ. Management of fever without source in infants and children. Ann Emerg Med 2000;36:602–14.
22. Warden CR, Zibulewsky J, Mace S, et al. Evaluation and management of febrile seizures in the out-of-hospital and emergency department settings. Ann Emerg Med 2003;41:215–22.

23. Ashkenazi S, Dinari G, Weitz R, et al. Convulsions in shigellosis. Evaluation of possible risk factors. Am J Dis Child 1983;137:985–7.
24. Kahn WA, Dhar U, Salam M, et al. Central nervous system manifestations of childhood shigellosis: prevalence, risk factors and outcome. Pediatrics 1999; 103:318.
25. Joffe A, McCormick M, DeAngelis C. Which children with febrile seizures need lumbar puncture? A decision analysis approach. Am J Dis Child 1983;137: 1153–6.
26. Soden J, Koch TK. Brain abscess presenting as a febrile seizure. Clin Pediatr 2000;39:365–8.
27. Kimia A, Ben-Joseph EP, Harper MB, et al. Yield of lumbar puncture among children who present with their first complex febrile seizure. Pediatrics 2010; 126:62–9.
28. Teng D, Dayan P, Hesdorffer D, et al. Risk of intracranial pathologic conditions requiring emergency intervention after a first complex febrile seizure episode among children. Pediatrics 2006;117:304–8.
29. Yucel O, Aka S, Yazicioglu L, et al. Role of early EEG and neuroimaging in determination of prognosis in children with complex febrile seizures. Pediatr Int 2004; 46:463–7.
30. Al-Qudah AA. Value of brain CT scan in children with febrile convulsions. J Neurol Sci 1995;128:107–10.
31. Offringa M, Bossuyt PM, Lubsen J, et al. Risk factors for seizure recurrence in children with febrile seizures: a pooled analysis of individual patient data from five studies. J Pediatr 1994;124:574–84.
32. Berg AT, Shinnar S, Darefsky AS, et al. Predictors of recurrent febrile seizures. A prospective cohort study. Arch Pediatr Adolesc Med 1997;151:371–8.
33. Schnaiderman D, Lahat E, Sheefer T, et al. Antipyretic effectiveness of acetaminophen in febrile seizures: ongoing prophylaxis versus sporadic usage. Eur J Pediatr 1993;152:747–9.
34. van Stuijvenberg M, Derksen-Lubsen G, Steyerberg EW, et al. Randomized, controlled trial of ibuprofen syrup administered during febrile illnesses to prevent febrile seizure recurrences. Pediatrics 1998;102:E51.
35. Van Esch A, Van Steensel-Moll HA, Steyerberg EW, et al. Antipyretic efficacy of ibuprofen and acetaminophen in children with febrile seizures. Arch Pediatr Adolesc Med 1995;149:632–7.
36. Strengell T, Uhari M, Tarkka R, et al. Antipyretic agents for preventing recurrences of febrile seizures. Arch Pediatr Adolesc Med 2009;163:799–804.
37. Uhari M, Rantala H, Vainionpaa L, et al. Effect of acetaminophen and of low intermittent doses of diazepam on prevention of recurrences of febrile seizures. J Pediatr 1995;126:991–5.
38. Schmitt BD. Fever phobia: misconceptions of parents about fevers. Am J Dis Child 1980;134:176–81.
39. Crocetti M, Moghbeli N, Serwint J. Fever phobia revisited: have parental misconceptions about fever changed in 20 years? Pediatrics 2001;107:1241–6.
40. van Stuijvenberg M, de Vos S, Tjiang GC, et al. Parents' fear regarding fever and febrile seizures. Acta Paediatr 1999;88:618–22.
41. Rosman NP, Colton T, Labazzo J, et al. A controlled trial of diazepam administered during febrile illnesses to prevent recurrence of febrile seizures. N Engl J Med 1993;329:79–84.
42. Knudsen FU. Recurrence risk after first febrile seizure and effect of short term diazepam prophylaxis. Arch Dis Child 1985;60:1045–9.

43. Ellenberg JH, Nelson KB. Febrile seizures and later intellectual performance. Arch Neurol 1978;35:17–21.
44. Norgaard M, Ehrenstein V, Mahon BE, et al. Febrile seizures and cognitive function in young adult life: a prevalence study in Danish conscripts. J Pediatr 2009;155:404–9.
45. Nelson KB, Ellenberg JH. Predisposing and causative factors in childhood epilepsy. Epilepsia 1987;28(Suppl 1):S16–24.

Afebrile Pediatric Seizures

Ghazala Q. Sharieff, MD[a,b], Phyllis L. Hendry, MD[c,*]

KEYWORDS

- Absence seizures • Neonatal seizures • Infantile spasms
- Afebrile • Hyponatremia • Convulsions • Epilepsy

Seizures in children can be anxiety provoking for both the parent and the medical caregiver. By 14 years of age, approximately 1% of children will experience an afebrile seizure with the highest incidence being in children younger than 3 years.[1] Population-based studies reveal that there are between 25,000 and 40,000 children per year in the United States who sustain a first-time, unprovoked seizure, 70% of which are idiopathic.[2,3] The overall recurrence rate in children with a first unprovoked afebrile seizure varies from 14% to 65%[4]; however, up to 88% of seizure recurrences occur within the first 2 years of the initial event.[5,6] Furthermore, Shinnar and colleagues[7] found that children who experience their first unprovoked seizure during sleep have approximately twice the recurrence rate as children whose first seizure occurred while awake. The first priority in a seizing patient is airway management and subsequent termination of the seizure.

SEIZURES THAT OCCUR IN CHILDHOOD
Absence Seizures

Simple (typical) absence seizures are uncommon before 5 years of age, and are typically characterized by a sudden cessation of motor activity with an accompanying

[a] Department of Emergency Medicine, Palomar-Pomerado Health System/California Emergency Physicians, 3020 Children's Way, San Diego, CA 92011, USA
[b] University of California, San Diego, CA, USA
[c] Department of Emergency Medicine, University of Florida College of Medicine, 655 West Eighth Street, Jacksonville, FL 32209, USA
* Corresponding author.
E-mail address: phyllis.hendry@jax.ufl.edu

Emerg Med Clin N Am 29 (2011) 95–108
doi:10.1016/j.emc.2010.08.009
0733-8627/11/$ – see front matter © 2011 Elsevier Inc. All rights reserved.

blank expression. Flickering of the eyelids may also be seen. The episodes last less than 30 seconds and are not associated with a postictal period. Complex (atypical) absence seizures are usually associated with myoclonic activity in the face or extremities, and are associated with an altered level of consciousness.

Lennox-Gastault

In this seizure disorder, patients experience a combination of tonic, absence, atonic, or myoclonic seizures with seizure onset between 3 and 5 years of age. Most of these children also have accompanying mental retardation and severe behavioral problems. An electroencephalogram (EEG) shows an irregular, slow, high-voltage spike pattern. While many drugs have been used to treat this condition, management is still very difficult. Valproic acid is the drug that is most commonly used; however, felbamate, topiramate, lamotrigine, and ethosuximide have also been used as add-on therapy.[8,9] The ketogenic diet (high fat, low protein, low carbohydrates) has been used with some success for these children. A study by Hemingway and colleagues[10] revealed that 13% of patients with intractable seizures who were treated with the ketogenic diet were seizure free at 1 year. Furthermore, a decrease by up to 99% in the frequency of seizures was noted in an additional 14% of patients who were started on the ketogenic diet. It is important to remember that if glucose is given, increased seizure activity may be seen.

Benign Rolandic Epilepsy

This syndrome typically involves children between 3 and 13 years of age who experience nighttime seizures. The initial phase of the seizure involves clonic activity of the face, which can then secondarily generalize. The history is characteristic with the seizures occurring during sleep. An EEG is important in the evaluation, as a characteristic perisylvian spiking pattern can be seen. Unless these seizures are frequent, no therapy is needed as patients will usually outgrow these episodes by early adulthood. Carbamazepine and levetiracetam have been used with success in the treatment of benign Rolandic seizures.

Juvenile Myoclonic Epilepsy of Janz

As the name implies, this disorder begins in early adolescence (peak age range is 12–15 years). Patients experience myoclonic jerks typically on awakening, but may also have tonic-clonic (80%) or absence (25%) seizures. Typical inducing factors include stress, alcohol, hormonal changes, or lack of sleep. The EEG is helpful in the diagnosis as a pattern of fast spike-and-wave discharges can be seen. Valproic acid has traditionally been the drug of choice; however, levetiracetam has shown effectiveness as both add-on and monotherapy for partial and generalized seizures.[1]

Infantile Spasms (West syndrome)

Children with this syndrome typically present between 4 and 18 months of age, and males are more commonly affected than females. Up to 95% of these children are mentally retarded and there is a 20% mortality rate. Patients experience spasms, which are typically single jerking episodes in flexion or extension of the involved muscle groups. The jerking is spasmodic, often occurring in clusters, and the child often cries during the episode. Episodes rarely occur during sleep. Up to 25% of patients have tuberous sclerosis. The EEG shows the classic pattern of hypsarrhythmia (random high-voltage slow waves with multifocal spikes). Treatment with adrenocorticotropic hormone (ACTH), prednisone vigabatrin, and pyridoxine have been used with some success. Valproic acid, lamotrigine, topiramate, zonisamide, levetiracetam, and benzodiazepines have also shown some effectiveness.[8,9,11,12]

EMERGENCY DEPARTMENT EVALUATION OF THE FIRST AFEBRILE SEIZURE
History and Physical Examination

The history should focus on the events immediately before the onset of the episode, a description of the seizure including seizure duration, cyanosis, loss of consciousness, the presence of incontinence, length of the postictal period, any postictal neurologic abnormalities, recent immunizations, change in diet or oral intake, and family history of seizures. A detailed birth history is important in new-onset seizures in neonates and infants. Home therapies and home remedies for any recent illnesses should also be determined. If the patient has a known seizure disorder, then it is important to ascertain if this seizure was different from previous seizures, the normal seizure frequency for the patient, medications the patient is on, if the patient has been compliant with the medication regimen, or if there have been any recent medication changes. The history may often help to differentiate a true seizure from a seizure mimic. Psychosocial history and recent family events are important in determining psychogenic seizures versus neurologic seizures. Patients who experience true seizures may describe an aura such as epigastric discomfort or a feeling of fear. The patient's positioning during the seizure, loss of sphincter control, duration of seizure, and the length of the postictal state should also be noted.

The physical examination focuses on the neurologic examination. In infants, measurement of head circumference may be helpful. A bulging fontanel indicates increased intracranial pressure. The eyes should be examined for papilledema and retinal hemorrhages. The presence of hepatosplenomegaly may indicate a metabolic or glycogen storage disease. The skin should also be checked for lesions such as café-au-lait spots (neurofibromatosis), vitiliginous lesions (tuberous sclerosis), and port-wine stains (Sturge-Weber syndrome). The differential diagnosis of seizures in children is listed in **Box 1**.

EMERGENCY DEPARTMENT MANAGEMENT

For the patient who is no longer seizing and whose airway is protected, little immediate management is needed beyond supportive care and continued monitoring. A bedside blood glucose reading should be obtained and hypoglycemia treated as follows: D_{10} solution (3–10 mL/kg) for newborns and D_{25} (2–4 mL/kg) solution for children. Dextrose should not be empirically given to children on ketogenic diets, as this will break the ketogenic state and may result in seizures. Any seizure that has lasted longer than 5 minutes should be treated with a benzodiazepine.[13] Lorazepam is an excellent choice, as it has an antiseizure duration of action of approximately 12 hours. Other options are diazepam and midazolam (**Table 1**). If the patient is actively seizing and intravenous (IV) access cannot be obtained, rectal diazepam, dosed at 0.3 to 0.5 mg/kg, can be administered.[15] Parents of known epileptics may have already administered this medication before paramedic arrival. Although diazepam has been the agent of choice in the past, recent studies support the use of midazolam.[16–18] The advantage of midazolam is that it can be administered by many routes including IV, intramuscular (IM), rectal, intranasal, and buccal.[19,20] In one study, when compared with IV diazepam, IM midazolam (0.2 mg/kg) resulted in faster seizure termination due to more rapid administration rates.[21]

Box 1
Differential diagnosis of seizures in children

Benign paroxysmal vertigo

Benign myoclonus of infancy

Benign sleep myoclonus

Breath-holding spells[a]

Gastroesophageal reflux

    Sandifer syndrome[b]

Migraine headaches

Night terrors, sleepwalking, somniloquy, narcolepsy[c]

Psychological

    Attention-deficit disorder

    Hyperventilation

    Hysteria and rage attacks

    Pseudoseizures

    Panic attacks

Shuddering attacks[d]

Sleepwalking

Syncope

Tics-Tourette syndrome

Toxins

[a] **Breath-holding spells:** Patients with cyanotic breath holding spells typically become angry, stop breathing in end-exhalation, pass out, and may have a hypoxic seizure.
[b] **Gastrointestinal reflux:** Infants with Sandifer syndrome present with crying, vomiting, esophagitis, and writhing and arching movements of the neck and back that may be confused with seizure activity.
[c] **Sleep disorders:** Night terrors occur when the child sits up suddenly during sleep, cries, screams, and is unresponsive to consoling attempts. The patient then returns to sleep and has no recollection of the event the next morning.
[d] **Paroxysmal movement disorders:** Shudder attacks are episodes of shivering activity that are not associated with any change in mental status. Spasmus mutans typically occurs in infants between 4 and 12 months of age, with the child experiencing head nodding, head tilt, and nystagmus.

If benzodiazepines do not terminate the seizure, the next agent of choice is either phenytoin or fosphenytoin because they do not cause central nervous system or respiratory depression. Fosphenytoin can be given 3 times as quickly as phenytoin (3 mg/kg/min vs 1 mg/kg/min) and reaches therapeutic serum concentrations within 15 minutes (phenytoin takes 25 minutes).[22]

LABORATORY TESTING

In patients who are on anticonvulsant medications, a drug level should be obtained. The practice of obtaining an electrolyte panel, and calcium and magnesium levels on every patient with a short seizure has been called into question in the child who

Table 1	
Drugs used in the management of seizures	
Diazepam	0.2–0.3 mg/kg IV, 0.5 mg/kg rectal
Lorazepam	0.05–0.1 mg/kg IV
Midazolam	0.1 mg/kg IV, 0.2 mg/kg IM
Phenytoin	15–20 mg/kg IV (no faster than 1 mg/kg/min)
Fosphenytoin	15–20 mg/kg IV or IM (can be given 3 mg/kg/min IV)
Phenobarbital	18–20 mg/kg IV, then 5–10 mg every 10 min (1 mg/kg/min) (maximum 50–60 mg/kg)
Levetiracetam	IV 50 mg/kg (maximum 2.5 g) Oral treatment should be initiated with a daily dose of 20 mg/kg in 2 divided doses (10 mg/kg bid). The daily dose should be increased every 2 weeks by increments of 20 mg/kg to the recommended daily dose of 60 mg/kg (30 mg/kg bid)[14]
Pyridoxine	50–100 mg IV
Lidocaine	1–2 mg/kg IV, then 4–6 mg/kg/h for refractory seizures

Abbreviations: bid, twice a day; IM, intramuscular; IV, intravenous.

is alert, interactive, and back to his or her baseline level of functioning. The Report of the Quality Standards Subcommittee of the American Academy of Neurology, the Child Neurology Society, and the American Epilepsy Society recommends that laboratory testing only be ordered based on clinical circumstances such as vomiting, diarrhea, dehydration, or failure to return to baseline level of consciousness.[23] Furthermore, a toxicology screen should be performed if there is any suspicion of drug exposure or abuse.

Newborns and children younger than 6 months have been found to be at greater risk for electrolyte abnormalities because of underlying metabolic abnormalities,[24] specifically hyponatremic seizures due to increased free water intake from formula overdilution. Farrar and colleagues[25] studied 47 patients younger than 6 months with seizures, and reported that the median seizure duration was longer (30 minutes vs 17 minutes, $P = .007$) in patients with hyponatremia, with a greater incidence of status epilepticus, 73% versus 36% ($P = .02$). Furthermore, emergency intubation was performed more often in hyponatremic patients than in normonatremic patients ($P = .009$). Median temperature was lower in hyponatremic infants (35.5°C vs 37.2°C, $P = .0001$). Temperature less than 36.5°C was the best predictor of hyponatremic seizures in infants younger than 6 months.

In a retrospective review of 149 infants younger than 12 months, Scarfone and colleagues[26] studied 214 visits for seizures, 80 of which were classified as febrile seizures. All laboratory results were reviewed: 19 of 80 febrile seizures were tested and none had abnormal electrolytes or calcium or magnesium levels: 67 of 134 non-febrile infants were tested, with 13% having abnormal chemistry results. However, patients with abnormal laboratory results were more likely to be actively seizing in the emergency department (ED), have hypothermia (temperature <36.5°C), or be younger than 1 month.

Based on the results of these studies, it is reasonable to obtain laboratory studies on pediatric patients with prolonged seizures, age less than 6 months, history of diabetes or metabolic disorder, dehydration or history of excess free water intake, and with an altered level of consciousness. Routine lumbar puncture in patients who are alert and oriented after a first afebrile seizure is not indicated. However, a spinal tap should be performed in patients with altered mental status, signs of meningitis/encephalitis, prolonged postictal period, or immunocompromised state, or if there is any suspicion of subarachnoid hemorrhage.

NEUROIMAGING

Magnetic resonance imaging (MRI) has superior resolution and is more sensitive than head computed tomography (CT) for the detection of low-grade tumors and heterotopic gray matter. A recent study of MRI findings in children with a first recognized seizure found at least one abnormality in 31% of children. Abnormalities defined as significant or related to seizures occurred in only 14%.[27] MRI is not readily available in all EDs and may be best performed on an outpatient nonemergent basis. MRI also lacks the radiation risks of CT scans.[28] Children are at greater risk than adults from a given dose of radiation because they are more radiosensitive and because they have more remaining years of life during which a radiation-induced cancer could develop.[29]

Although many providers routinely perform CT scans on every patient with new-onset seizures, this practice has been called into question. In 1997, Warden and colleagues[30] recommended that emergent neuroimaging be reserved for patients with a prolonged postictal period, status epilepticus, age less than 6 months, new-onset focal neurologic defects, recent head injury, patients with ventriculoperitoneal shunts, or other neurocutaneous disorders. In 1998, Garvey and colleagues[31] conducted a retrospective analysis of 107 neurologically normal patients who underwent neuroimaging in the ED for "first seizure": 8 of 107 had nonepileptic events (gastroesophageal reflux, syncope, and rigor). Of the remaining 99 patients, 49 had provoked seizures and 50 had unprovoked seizures: 19 of 99 patients had CT abnormalities, and 9 of 49 with provoked seizures had abnormalities on CT, but none required intervention (mild hydrocephalus, angioma, asymmetry, periventricular leukomalacia). Ten of 50 patients with unprovoked seizures had CT abnormalities, with 7 receiving further investigation or interventions: 2 had tumors, 3 had vascular abnormalities, 1 had cysticercosis, and 1 had obstructive hydrocephalus. In this study, CT scan abnormalities requiring treatment or monitoring were more often seen in children with unprovoked seizures ($P<.01$) and in children with focal seizures or focal neurologic findings ($P<.04$).

Sharma and colleagues[32] reviewed 500 patients with new-onset seizures, of whom 475 underwent neuroimaging. The mean patient age was 62 months (range 0–21 months). Focal seizures were present in 33% of patients. Risk factors for neuroimaging abnormalities included the presence of a predisposing condition or a focal seizure in children younger than 33 months. Predisposing conditions were sickle cell disease, bleeding disorders, cerebral vascular disease, malignancy, human immunodeficiency virus (HIV), hydrocephalus, travel to areas with cysticercosis, closed head injury, or the presence of hemihypertrophy. Clinically significant findings were present in 8% (38/475) of patients who underwent neuroimaging. Twenty-six percent (32/121) of high-risk patients had abnormalities versus 2% (6/354) of the low-risk patients. The investigators concluded that emergent imaging should be performed only in patients with high-risk criteria. Furthermore, they advised that if follow-up can be obtained, low-risk patients can be discharged without immediate ED imaging.

A practice guideline written jointly by the Quality Standards Subcommittee of the American Academy of Neurology, the Child Neurology Society, and the American Epilepsy Society concur that there is insufficient evidence to support the routine performance of neuroimaging in children with a first unprovoked nonfebrile seizure.[23]

Bedside brain ultrasonography is often the imaging study of choice in neonatal seizures, due to challenges of transporting critically ill neonates to CT or MRI. The disadvantage of ultrasonography is the poor detection of cortical lesions and subarachnoid blood.

ELECTROENCEPHALOGRAPHY

An EEG is rarely needed in the ED setting, except for patients with refractory seizures or in patients in whom the diagnosis of nonconvulsive status epilepticus is being considered. Well-appearing children who have experienced a first-time afebrile seizure can be managed as outpatients, with an EEG arranged by the primary care physician. In idiopathic and cryptogenic seizures, the EEG has been found to be the most important predictor of recurrence, with a 2-year recurrence rate of 58% in patients with an abnormal EEG compared with a 28% seizure recurrence rate in patients with a normal EEG.[33] Of note, a normal EEG does not rule out a seizure disorder or other underlying neurologic disorder.

Portable EEG monitoring is now available in many EDs and pediatric intensive care units, and can be used to determine treatment response.

ANTIEPILEPTIC AGENTS

In a critical review of the literature, the Quality Standards Subcommittee of the American Academy of Neurology and the Practice Committee of the Child Neurology Society found that although anticonvulsant agents decrease the incidence of second seizures, they do not decrease the long-term risk of developing epilepsy.[23] Therefore, they recommend that for stable, well-appearing children who have experienced a single seizure that did not require emergent anticonvulsant therapy, maintenance medications are not initiated. Patients who experience recurrent seizures should be started on an antiepileptic medication. The decision to initiate long-term anticonvulsant therapy should be made in conjunction with a pediatric neurologist or the patient's primary care physician. The most common agents used to treat afebrile seizures are listed in **Table 2**. Felbamate is not commonly used because of the availability of safer antiepileptic agents, and is indicated only for cases of severe refractory seizures (Lennox-Gastault syndrome) where the benefit clearly outweighs the risk of liver toxicity and aplastic anemia.

NEONATAL SEIZURES

It is often difficult in the newborn to differentiate between a seizure from other conditions, especially because newborn seizures can present in a variety of different ways including apnea, subtle eye deviations, or abnormal chewing movements. In addition, associated autonomic system findings seen with older patients with seizures may not be seen. Useful tips in differentiating between a newborn with seizures and a "jittery baby" are that true seizures cannot be suppressed by passive restraint and seizures cannot be elicited by motion or startling.

The most common cause of a seizure in the first 3 days of life is perinatal hypoxia or anoxia. Approximately 50% to 65% of newborn seizures are due to hypoxic-ischemic encephalopathy.[34] Intraventricular, subdural, and subarachnoid hemorrhages account for 15% of newborn seizures, and an additional 10% are caused by inborn errors of metabolism, sepsis, metabolic disorders, and toxins (**Box 2**).[35] Pyridoxine deficiency is an autosomal recessive disorder that is a rare cause of seizures, and usually presents in the first 1 to 2 days of life.[36]

Benign familial neonatal convulsions and benign idiopathic neonatal convulsions are 2 types of neonatal seizures that are benign and carry a favorable prognosis.

Table 2
Common anticonvulsant agents

Drug	Type of Seizure	Side Effects	Maintenance
Carbamazepine (Tegretol)	Generalized tonic-clonic, partial, benign Rolandic seizures	Rash, liver disease, diplopia, aplastic anemia, leukopenia	10–40 mg/kg divided bid or tid
Clonazepam (Rivotril, Klonopin)	Myoclonic, akinetic, infantile spasms, partial, Lennox-Gastault	Fatigue, behavioral issues, salivation	0.05–0.3 mg/kg/d divided bid or tid
Ethosuximide (Zarontin)	Absence	GI upset, weight gain, lethargy, SLE, rash	20–40 mg/kg/d divided qd or bid
Gabapentin (Neurontin)	Partial and secondarily generalized seizures	Fatigue, dizziness, diarrhea, ataxia	20–70 mg/kg/d
Lamotrigine (Lamictal)	Complex partial (atypical absence), Lennox-Gastaut, myoclonic, absence, tonic-clonic	Headache, nausea, rash, Stevens-Johnson syndrome, lymphadenopathy, diplopia, GI upset	10–12 mg/kg/d if given as monotherapy, 2–5 mg/kg/d if given with valproic acid
Levetiracetam (Keppra)	Partial-onset seizures in children >4 y, generalized tonic-clonic seizures in children >6 y, juvenile myoclonic seizures in children >12 y	Dizziness, somnolence, headache	20 mg/kg/d divided bid. Daily dose increased every 2 wk by increments of 20 mg/kg to the recommended daily dose of 60 mg/kg (30 mg/kg bid)
Phenobarbital (Luminol)	Generalized tonic-clonic, partial	Sedation, behavioral issues	2–6 mg/kg/d divided qd or bid
Phenytoin (Dilantin)	Generalized tonic-clonic, partial	Gingival hyperplasia, hirsutism, rash, Stevens-Johnson syndrome, lymphoma	4–8 mg/kg/d divided bid, tid, or qhs

Drug	Indication	Side effects	Dosage
Primidone (Mysoline)	Generalized tonic-clonic, partial	Rash, ataxia, behavioral issues, sedation, anemia	10–25 mg/kg/d divided bid, tid, or qid
Topiramate (Topamax)	Refractory complex partial seizures, infantile spasms, adjunctive therapy for temporal lobe epilepsy	Fatigue, nephrolithiasis, ataxia, headache, tremor, GI upset	1–9 mg/kg/d
Tiagabine (Gabitril)	Adjunctive therapy for refractory complex partial (focal) seizures	Decreased attention span, tremor, dizziness, anorexia	Average dose 6 mg/d
Valproic acid (Epicene, Epical)	Generalized tonic-clonic, absence, myoclonic, partial, akinetic, juvenile myoclonic epilepsy of Janz, infantile spasms	GI upset, liver involvement, alopecia, sedation	10–60 mg/kg/d divided tid or qid
Vigabatrin (Sabril)	Infantile spasms, adjunctive therapy for refractory seizures	Weight gain, agitation, depression, behavioral changes, visual field constriction, optic neuritis	30–100 mg/kg/d divided qd or bid
Oxcarbazepine (Trileptal)	Partial/focal seizures	Hyponatremia, hepatic or blood dyscrasias	20–40 mg/kg/d
Zonis amide (zonegran)	Adjunctive therapy for partial or general seizures	Rash, renal calculi, photosensitivity	Begin with 1–2 mg/kg/d

Abbreviations: bid, twice a day; GI, gastrointestinal; SLE, systemic lupus erythematosus; tid, 3 times a day; qd, every day; qhs, every bedtime; qid, 4 times a day.

Box 2
Etiology of newborn seizures

First day of life

    Anoxia

    Hypoxia

    Trauma

    Intracranial hemorrhage

    Drugs

    Infection

    Hypoglycemia/hyperglycemia

    Pyridoxine deficiency

Second and third day of life

    Sepsis

    Inborn errors of metabolism

    Trauma

    Hypocalcemia

    Hypoglycemia

    Hypomagnesemia

    Hyperphosphatemia

    Hyponatremia/hypernatremia

    Drug withdrawal

    Congenital anomalies

    Developmental brain disorders

    Benign familial neonatal seizures

    Hypertension

Day 4 of life to 6 months of age

    Hypocalcemia

    Hyponatremia/hypernatremia

    Infection

    Drug withdrawal

    Inborn errors of metabolism

    Hyperphosphatemia

    Hypertension

    Congenital anomalies

    Developmental brain disorders

    Benign idiopathic neonatal seizures

The etiology is unknown. Benign familial neonatal convulsions typically present in the first 3 days of life, and there is a strong family history of epilepsy or neonatal seizures. These seizures resolve by 1 to 6 months of age. Benign idiopathic neonatal convulsions, also known as "fifth-day fits," occur on the fifth day of life and cease on day 15 of life.[36] These diagnoses should be ones of exclusion. The workup should be tailored to the patient but may include cranial ultrasonography, a head CT or MRI scan, electrolytes, glucose, calcium, magnesium, toxicology screen, urinalysis and culture, complete blood count and culture, and cerebrospinal fluid (CSF) studies. If an inborn error of metabolism is suspected, then blood for amino acids, lactate, pyruvate and ammonia levels should be obtained, as well as urine for organic acids.

In neonates who are actively seizing, treatment includes attention to the airway, breathing, and circulation. Benzodiazepines are often given as the first line of treatment, followed by phenobarbital, fosphenytoin, or phenytoin, all of which have risks and benefits.[34] Benzodiazepines have been associated with serious adverse effects such as hypotension and respiratory depression in preterm and term infants, and therefore should be used with caution.[37] Phenytoin is not the preferred initial agent, as it has a depressive effect on the newborn myocardium and has an unpredictable rate of metabolism due to immature hepatic function.[33] Pyridoxine (50–100 mg IV) or lidocaine may be used if refractory seizures are present (see **Table 1**).[36] If the seizure is a result of an electrolyte abnormality such as hyponatremia, hypocalcemia, or hypomagnesemia, these abnormalities should be rapidly identified and treated. In patients who are actively seizing, hyponatremia can be treated with normal saline (0.9%) boluses or alternatively with 5 to 10 mL/kg IV of 3% saline (this can be administered as a bolus given over 10 minutes). If the patient has hypocalcemia (plasma calcium <7.0 mg/dL), then 100 to 300 mg/kg of IV 10% calcium gluconate should be infused. In cases of hypomagnesemia (serum magnesium <1 mEq/L), 0.1 to 0.3 mL/kg of 50% magnesium sulfate should be given IV IV or IM. Ampicillin and cefotaxime should be initiated in any patient considered to have sepsis. Acyclovir (20 mg/kg every 8 h IV) should also be administered if there is a positive maternal history of herpes, if the patient has a vesicular rash, focal neurologic findings, or a CSF pleocytosis or elevated CSF protein without organisms on Gram stain.[38] Patients should be admitted to a monitored bed for further observation and evaluation.

FUTURE DIRECTIONS

Future research needs must focus on:

- Neuroimaging safety and guidelines for imaging
- Safe antiepileptic drugs for children
- Improved access to pediatric neurologic evaluation for the subset of children with difficult to manage and refractory afebrile seizures.

SUMMARY

Afebrile seizures in children are common and often recur. Fortunately, most children with childhood epilepsy have a favorable long-term prognosis. In particular, patients with idiopathic etiology usually reach remission.[39] There are specific types of afebrile seizure disorders that emergency physicians should be aware of, with absence seizures being the most common. Newborn seizures are often difficult to diagnose, and are evaluated and treated more aggressively than afebrile seizures in older infants and children. Children that present to the ED often have a known seizure disorder, are taking medications for their disorder, and usually are in a postictal state on arrival. Seizures lasting longer than 5 minutes should be treated initially with a benzodiazepine and standard advanced life support protocols. Laboratory studies are needed only in children younger than 6 months, in patients with prolonged seizures or altered level of consciousness, or in patients with history of a metabolic disorder or dehydration. Routine neuroimaging is not recommended in children with a first unprovoked afebrile seizure, although imaging studies should be considered in children younger than 3 years with a predisposing condition or focal seizures. Most well-appearing children can be managed as outpatients after a first afebrile seizure, with instructions for an outpatient EEG and follow-up by the primary care physician. Anticonvulsant drugs do not decrease the long-term incidence of epilepsy and are therefore not usually recommended after a first afebrile seizure. New anticonvulsant drugs continue to be investigated, but it is important to recognize that no anticonvulsive agents decrease the long-term incidence of epilepsy and are therefore not usually recommended after a first afebrile seizure. Adjunct nonpharmacologic therapies such as vagal nerve stimulation are also being used in patients with severe epilepsy. Intermittent electrical stimulation is delivered to the cervical vagus nerve. The lead is usually located on the left side of the neck, and the generator is implanted in the chest wall. The emergency provider should keep abreast of new technologies and emerging trends in pharmacologic antiepileptic management.

KEY CONCEPTS

- An EEG should be performed as soon as possible on patients with an apparent first unprovoked seizure.
- Electrolyte testing is not routinely necessary on well-appearing children older than 6 months.
- Emergent neuroimaging of children with first-time seizures should be performed on patients with the following risk factors: focal seizures, prolonged postictal period, status epilepticus, sickle cell disease, immunocompromise, head injury, age less than 6 months to 1 year, ventriculoperitoneal shunts, recent travel to an area endemic for cysticercosis, bleeding disorders, cerebral vascular disease, neurocutaneous disorders, malignancy, HIV, or hydrocephalus.
- Well-appearing children who have experienced a first unprovoked seizure and are in the low-risk category do not need emergent neuroimaging if they have close outpatient follow-up.
- Children on ketogenic diets should not be given dextrose empirically.

REFERENCES

1. Verrotti A, D'Adamo E, Parisi P, et al. Levetiracetam in childhood epilepsy. Paediatr Drugs 2010;12(3):177–86.
2. Camfield CS, Camfield PR, Gordon K, et al. Incidence of epilepsy in childhood and adolescence: a population-based study in Nova Scotia from 1977 to 1985. Epilepsia 1996;37(1):19–23.
3. Hauser WA, Annegers JF, Kurland LT. Incidence of epilepsy and unprovoked seizures in Rochester, Minnesota: 1935–1984. Epilepsia 1993;34(3):453–68.
4. Hirtz D, Berg A, Bettis D, et al. Practice parameter: treatment of the child with a first unprovoked seizure: report of the quality standards subcommittee of the American Academy of Neurology and the Practice Committee of the Child Neurology Society. Neurology 2003;60(2):166–75.
5. Shinnar S, Berg AT, O'Dell C, et al. Predictors of multiple seizures in a cohort of children prospectively followed from the time of their first unprovoked seizure. Ann Neurol 2000;48(2):140–7.

6. Stroink H, Brouwer OF, Arts WF, et al. The first unprovoked, untreated seizure in childhood: a hospital based study of the accuracy of the diagnosis, rate of recurrence, and long term outcome after recurrence. Dutch study of epilepsy in childhood. J Neurol Neurosurg Psychiatry 1998;64(5):595–600.

7. Shinnar S, Berg AT, Ptachewich Y, et al. Sleep state and the risk of seizure recurrence following a first unprovoked seizure in childhood. Neurology 1993;43(4):701–6.

8. Trevathan E. Infantile spasms and Lennox-Gastaut syndrome. J Child Neurol 2002;17(Suppl 2):2S9–22.

9. Hancodk EC, Osborne JP, Edwards SW. Treatment of infantile spasms. Cochrane Database Syst Rev 2008;4:CD001770.

10. Hemingway C, Freeman JM, Pillas DJ. The ketogenic diet: a 3- to 6-year follow-up of 150 children enrolled prospectively. Pediatrics 2001;108(4): 898–905.

11. Cossette P, Riviello JJ, Carmant L. ACTH versus vigabatrin therapy in infantile spasms: a retrospective study. Neurology 1999;52(8):1691–4.

12. Elterman RD, Shields WD, Mansfield KA, et al. Randomized trial of vigabatrin in patients with infantile spasms. Neurology 2001;57(8):1416–21.

13. Lowenstein DH, Alldredge BK. Status epilepticus. N Engl J Med 1998;338(14): 970–6.

14. Ng YT, Hastriter EV, Cardenas JF, et al. Intravenous levetiracetam in children with seizures: a prospective safety study. J Child Neurol 2010;25(5):551–5.

15. Fitzgerald BJ, Okos AJ, Miller JW. Treatment of out-of-hospital status epilepticus with diazepam rectal gel. Seizure 2003;12(1):52–5.

16. Rainbow J, Browne GJ, Lam LT. Controlling seizures in the prehospital setting: diazepam or midazolam? J Paediatr Child Health 2002;38(6):582–6.

17. Chamberlain JM, Altieri MA, Futterman C, et al. A prospective, randomized study comparing intramuscular midazolam with intravenous diazepam for the treatment of seizures in children. Pediatr Emerg Care 1997;13(2):92–4.

18. Vilke GM, Sharieff GQ, Marino A, et al. Midazolam for the treatment of out-of-hospital pediatric seizures. Prehosp Emerg Care 2002;6(2):215–7.

19. Ashrafi MR, Khosroshahi N, Karimi P. Efficacy and usability of buccal midazolam in controlling acute prolonged convulsive seizures in children. Eur J Paediatr Neurol 2010;14(5):434–8.

20. Scott RC, Besag FM, Neville BG. Buccal midazolam and rectal diazepam for treatment of prolonged seizures in childhood and adolescence: a randomised trial. Lancet 1999;353(9153):623–6.

21. Gottwald MD, Akers LC, Liu PK, et al. Prehospital stability of diazepam and lorazepam. Am J Emerg Med 1999;17(4):333–7.

22. Fischer JH, Patel TV, Fischer PA. Fosphenytoin: clinical pharmacokinetics and comparative advantages in the acute treatment of seizures. Clin Pharmacokinet 2003;42(1):33–58.

23. Hirtz D, Ashwal S, Berg A, et al. Practice parameter: evaluating a first nonfebrile seizure in children: report of the quality standards subcommittee of the American Academy of Neurology, The Child Neurology Society, and The American Epilepsy Society. Neurology 2000;55(5):616–23.

24. Bui TT, Delgado CA, Simon HK. Infant seizures not so infantile: first-time seizures in children under six months of age presenting to the ED. Am J Emerg Med 2002; 20(6):518–20.

25. Farrar HC, Chande VT, Fitzpatrick DF, et al. Hyponatremia as the cause of seizures in infants: a retrospective analysis of incidence, severity, and clinical predictors. Ann Emerg Med 1995;26(1):42–8.

26. Scarfone RJ, Pond K, Thompson K, et al. Utility of laboratory testing for infants with seizures. Pediatr Emerg Care 2000;16(5):309–12.

27. Kalnin AJ, Fastenau PS, deGrauw TJ, et al. Magnetic resonance imaging findings in children with a first recognized seizure. Pediatr Neurol 2008;39: 404–14.

28. Gaillard WD, Chiron C, Cross JH, et al. Guidelines for imaging infants and children with recent-onset epilepsy. Epilepsia 2009;50:2147–53.

29. Brenner DJ, Hall EJ. Computed tomography—an increasing source of radiation exposure. N Engl J Med 2007;357(22):2277–84.

30. Warden CR, Brownstein DR, Del Beccaro MA. Predictors of abnormal findings of computed tomography of the head in pediatric patients presenting with seizures. Ann Emerg Med 1997;29(4):518–23.

31. Garvey MA, Gaillard WD, Rusin JA, et al. Emergency brain computed tomography in children with seizures: who is most likely to benefit? J Pediatr 1998; 133(5):664–9.

32. Sharma S, Riviello JJ, Harper MB, et al. The role of emergent neuroimaging in children with new-onset afebrile seizures. Pediatrics 2003;111(1):1–5.

33. Shinnar S, Berg AT, Moshe SL, et al. The risk of seizure recurrence after a first unprovoked afebrile seizure in childhood: an extended follow-up. Pediatrics 1996;98(2 Pt 1):216–25.

34. Stafstrom CE. Neonatal seizures. Pediatr Rev 1995;16(7):248–55.

35. Bernes SM, Kaplan AM. Evolution of neonatal seizures. Pediatr Clin North Am 1994;41(5):1069–104.

36. Evans D, Levene M. Neonatal seizures. Arch Dis Child Fetal Neonatal Ed 1998; 78(1):F70–5.

37. Ng E, Klinger G, Shah V, et al. Safety of benzodiazepines in newborns. Ann Pharmacother 2002;36(7–8):1150–5.

38. Riley LE. Herpes simplex virus. Semin Perinatol 1998;22(4):284–92.

39. Geerts A, Arts WF, Stroink H, et al. Course and outcome of childhood epilepsy: a 15-year follow-up of the Dutch study of epilepsy in childhood. Epilepsia 2010;51:1189–97.

Seizures in Pregnancy/Eclampsia

Latha Ganti Stead, MD, MS[a,b,*]

KEYWORDS

• Seizure • Pregnancy • Pre-eclampsia • Eclampsia

Seizures in pregnancy can be classified into three categories: (1) those that can occur independent of the pregnant state, (2) those that are exacerbated by the pregnant state, and (3) those that are unique to the pregnant state. Seizures in the first category, that is, those that are not specifically related with the pregnant state are covered elsewhere in this issue of *Emergency Medicine Clinics of North America* and therefore will not be discussed in this article. The goals of this article are to answer the following questions:

What is the pathophysiology of preeclampsia?
How are eclamptic seizures best managed?
What are the implications of seizures for the mother and child?

SEIZURES AND PREGNANCY

Most patients seen in the emergency department who have a seizure in pregnancy have a known seizure disorder and are on an antiepileptic drug (AED). The choice and dose of the AED usually are managed by the primary care physician. All AEDs have been linked to some teratogenic effect, so the risks versus benefits must be weighed.[1] Phenytoin and carbamazepine are the drugs most commonly used, and of the two, carbamazepine is preferred. Valproic acid is reported to reduce cognitive outcome at age 3, independent of maternal IQ. This effect also has been reported for phenytoin and carbamazepine.[2] Phenobarbital is also used, albeit less commonly.

Total blood levels of an AED will tend to go down during the pregnancy due to an increase in hepatic and renal clearance of the drug, and a pregnancy-related increase in the volume of distribution of the drug.[3–5] This decrease in serum drug level is balanced by the fact that free (unbound) drug levels may actually be increased due to the decrease in concentration of serum proteins that normally occurs in pregnancy.

[a] Division of Clinical Research, Department of Emergency Medicine, University of Florida College of Medicine, 1329 SW 16th Street, Gainesville, FL 32610, USA
[b] Department of Emergency Medicine, Mayo Clinic College of Medicine, 200 First Street SW, Rochester, MN 55905, USA
* Division of Clinical Research, Department of Emergency Medicine, University of Florida College of Medicine, 1329 SW 16th Street, Gainesville, FL 32610.
E-mail address: lstead@ufl.edu

Emerg Med Clin N Am 29 (2011) 109–116
doi:10.1016/j.emc.2010.09.005
0733-8627/11/$ – see front matter © 2011 Elsevier Inc. All rights reserved.

Because serum drug levels depend on several factors, and the physiology of pregnancy changes from month to month, epileptic patients usually have their AED levels monitored monthly and have their AED dose(s) adjusted accordingly.

The most common cause for seizures in pregnant women with a known seizure disorder is noncompliance with medication. This often has to do with misconceptions that the patient may have regarding potential teratogenicity of the AED(s); patients should be educated about the risk of seizure and status epilepticus on the fetus, and the importance of compliance should be emphasized.

Other factors that may lower the seizure threshold in pregnancy include sleep deprivation, nausea and vomiting, and subsequent dehydration. Ideally patients with seizure disorders plan their pregnancies, and have taken the time to devise a good AED regimen with their primary care doctor, as well as get other things in life organized in such a way as to cause the least stress. The Australian Pregnancy Registry[6] reports that epileptic women who have been seizure free in the year before becoming pregnant had a 50% to 70% smaller risk of seizing during the pregnancy.

The management of seizures in pregnancy is the same as for any nonpregnant patient. The main difference is the importance of supplemental oxygen. Hypoxia is not a major concern for most seizing patients; however, it is a serious risk to the fetus.

PREECLAMPSIA

Eclampsia is a condition that manifests with seizures that is unique to the pregnant state. Patients have an underlying condition known as preeclampsia, or pregnancy-induced hypertension (PIH). Preeclampsia complicates 2% to 8% of all pregnancies,[7] and is characterized classically by the triad of hypertension, proteinuria, and edema. More recently, edema has been eliminated as a diagnostic criterion, as many pregnant women have edema as part of their pregnancy without ever developing preeclampsia. The proteinuria is defined as greater than 0.3 g over a 24 hour collection period. This corresponds roughly to 1+ on commercial urine dipsticks. Gestational blood pressure elevation is defined as a blood pressure greater than 140 mm Hg systolic or 90 mm Hg diastolic in a woman who was normotensive before 20 weeks gestation. It is important to note that hypertension in this case is relative, as a blood pressure of 140/90 may be hypertensive for a pregnant woman in the first trimester, when blood pressure is physiologically lower. Women are routinely screened for proteinuria and high blood pressure in an effort to detect preeclampsia. Even in the absence of proteinuria, (which may not yet be manifest), preeclampsia is highly suspect if in addition to hypertension, there are symptoms of headache, blurred vision, or abdominal pain. Laboratory parameters that support the diagnosis or development of preeclampsia include thrombocytopenia, elevated liver function tests, and evidence of microangiopathic hemolytic anemia (elevated serum lactate dehydrogenase, decreased serum haptoglobin, presence of schistocytes on peripheral smear). Hemoconcentration also is noted frequently. Preeclampsia can progress to the fulminate HELLP syndrome, characterized by (hemolysis, elevated liver enzymes, and low platelet counts), which increases the risk of adverse maternal and fetal outcomes. Elevated uric acid levels greater than 6 also can be a marker of disease, with a positive predictive value of 33%.

Risk factors for preeclampsia include extremes of maternal age, nulliparity, a family history of preeclampsia or eclampsia, multiple gestations, pregestational diabetes, renal disease, and trophoblastic diseases such as fetal hydrops and hydatiform mole. Women who develop signs of preeclampsia before 20 weeks should be evaluated for the presence of a hydatiform mole, a pseudopregnant state that carries a risk of choriocarcinoma.

ECLAMPSIA

Eclampsia is defined as seizures in a woman with preeclampsia that cannot be attributed to any other cause. Patients often will show signs of preeclampsia starting at about 20 to 24 weeks. About a quarter of eclampsia-related seizures occur before labor. About a half occur during labor, and another quarter occur postpartum, up to 10 days out. The seizures in eclampsia are thought to be secondary to hypertensive encephalopathy.[8]

Pathophysiology of Eclampsia

Despite the prevalence of the problem and the numerous clinical trials, the exact underlying etiology for the disease has yet to be elucidated. The end result in preeclampsia is widespread endothelial dysfunction in the mother, presumed to be secondary to either genetic susceptibility or a maladaptive immune system, which is ultimately responsible for the hypertension, microangiopathic hemolytic anemia, edema, and other clinical manifestations seen. The pathophysiology also involves abnormal migration of trophoblastic cells early in the pregnancy (well before clinical signs are apparent), resulting in poor placental perfusion. This poor perfusion is exacerbated in situations where there are increased demands on the placentofetal unit, such as in multiple gestations, and fetal macrosomia. Additionally, platelet function is disturbed in preeclampsia. Quantitatively, there are less of them (thrombocytopenia), and qualitatively, they have a shorter lifespan (increased hemolysis).

Management of Eclampsia

Seizure control

The immediate goals in the management of eclampsia are to stop the current seizure and prevent recurrence of seizures. The two drugs most commonly used are magnesium sulfate and phenytoin. A systematic review of four good-quality trials involving 823 women found magnesium sulfate to be substantially more effective than phenytoin, with regards to recurrence of convulsions (relative risk [RR] 0.32, 95% confidence interval [CI] 0.21–0.50) and maternal death (RR 0.5, 95% CI 0.24–1.05]).[8] Complications such as respiratory depression (RR 0.71, 95% CI 0.46–1.09]) and pneumonia (RR 0.44,95% CI 0.24–0.79) were also less for magnesium than for phenytoin. Magnesium showed a trend toward increased incidence of renal failure when compared with phenytoin (RR 1.42, 95% CI 0.90–2.26), but this was not statistically significant. Magnesium sulfate also was associated with benefits for the baby, including fewer admissions to the neonatal intensive care unit (NICU) (RR 0.73, 95% CI 0.58–0.91) and fewer babies who died or were in the NICU for more than 7 days (RR 0.77, 95% CI 0.63–0.95). A separate systematic review looked at treatment of preeclampsia with magnesium sulfate versus placebo or no anticonvulsant, and found that magnesium sulfate halved the risk of eclampsia (RR 0.41, 95% CI 0.29–0.58), with a number needed to treat (NNT) of 100 (95% CI 50–100).[9] It also reduced the risk of placental abruption (RR 0.64, 95% CI 0.50–0.83), with an NNT of 100 (95% CI 50–1000). The risk of maternal death also was reduced by magnesium, although this was not statistically significant. On the negative side, treatment with magnesium sulfate also resulted in a small increase (approximately 5%) in frequency of delivery by cesarean section. Approximately 25% of women experienced flushing as a side effect of magnesium.

The mechanism of action of magnesium involves generalized central nervous system (CNS) depression, which serves to attenuate seizures. Dilation of the cerebral arteries serves to rescue brain ischemia. Magnesium also has tocolytic activity and a mild antihypertensive effect. The usual dose is a 4 g bolus that is repeated until seizures stop. It can then be given as an infusion at a rate of 1–3 g/h for at least 24 hours. Therapeutic range is between 4–5 mEq/L. The adverse effects include flushing (benign) and respiratory depression, which are usually seen at serum levels of >10 mEq/L. The first clinical sign of magnesium toxicity is loss of deep tendon reflexes. Therefore, serial neurologic examinations are imperative in patients receiving magnesium therapy. Magnesium overdose is treated with 10% calcium gluconate or chloride solution and cardiorespiratory support.

Blood Pressure Control

After seizure control, the next major parameter to control in eclampsia is hypertension. Agents of choice per the American College of Obstetrics and Gynecology (ACOG) and the National High Blood Pressure Education Program: Working Group Report on High Blood Pressure in Pregnancy include hydralazine (first-line) and labetalol.[10] In resistant cases, nitroprusside also may be used, although fetal cyanide toxicity can occur after a few hours of therapy. Oral nifedipine has been advocated by some, but it is not approved by the US Food and Drug Administration (FDA) for this indication. Generally, treatment of blood pressure is instituted for systolic blood pressure greater than 160 mm Hg or diastolic blood pressure greater than 105 mm Hg. **Table 1** summarizes the antihypertensive regimens.

A systematic review of 1637 women concluded that there is no good evidence that any one antihypertensive is better than the other with regard to outcomes of eclampsia,

Table 1
Antihypertensive regimens for preeclampsia and eclampsia

Drug	Initial Bolus	Subsequent Dosing	Caveats/Notes
Hydralazine	10–20 mg intravenously or 20 mg intramuscularly	Repeat bolus if no response in 20 min Consider another drug if no response after 3 boluses If response achieved, repeat bolus every 3 hours	Onset of action is 20 min Adverse effects include headache, flushing, lightheadedness, nausea, palpitations
Labetalol	20 mg intravenous bolus	If no response or suboptimal response, give 2nd bolus of 40 mg 10 min later If still suboptimal response can escalate dose to 80 mg bolus 10 min apart, for a maximum dose of 220 mg total Once response is achieved, can maintain on infusion of 1 mg/kg	Contraindicated in 2nd and 3rd degree heart block and severe asthma Adverse effects include flushing, lightheadedness, scalp tingling
Nitroprusside		Start at a rate of 0.3 μg/kg/min Titrate to effect Maximum dose is 5 μg/kg/min	Watch out for fetal cyanide toxicity

cesarean section, maternal side effects, persistent maternal hypertension, or fetal/neonatal death.[11] The antihypertensives included in this review were hydralazine, calcium channel blockers (nifedipine, nimodipine, nicardipine, and isradipine), labetalol, methyldopa, diazoxide, prostacyclin, ketanserin, urapidil, magnesium sulfate, prazosin, and isosorbide. Interestingly, diazoxide was significantly associated with hypotension, while ketanserin failed to lower the blood pressure effectively. For this reason, neither of these drugs is recommended for use in preeclampsia or eclampsia. Interestingly, no randomized controlled trials studying nitroprusside for preeclampsia have been published, despite it being one of the recommended (albeit not first-line) regimens.

Plasma Volume Expansion

The rationale for the plasma volume expansion in the treatment of preeclampsia is that the blood volume fails to expand with the pregnancy as it should. A systematic review of three trials involving 61 women compared administration of colloid solution versus no plasma volume expansion, and found insufficient evidence to support its use.[12] No randomized clinical trials using crystalloid for plasma expansion were published at the time of the review.

Diuretics

Diuretics have been used in preeclampsia under the rationale that they reduce edema and blood pressure, two of the hallmarks of the disease. However, concern arose over the plasma volume reduction that diuretics also cause. A Cochrane review of five studies including 1836 women put the debate to rest.[13] While no clear harm was demonstrated with diuretic use with regard to the outcomes of preeclampsia, preterm birth, or perinatal death, no clear benefits were found with diuretic use either. This finding, taken together with the known adverse effects of nausea and vomiting, result in the recommendation they not be used for the prevention of preeclampsia.

The Ultimate Care

The definitive treatment for eclampsia is delivery of the fetus. If the patient is at term, or the fetus is of an age where viability is not a concern, the decision is not difficult. In situations where the fetus is less than at term, maternal health and the viability of the fetus in utero (with its inherent risks) versus in the nursery must be weighted. **Box 1** outlines indications where emergent delivery should be considered. A systematic review[8] involving 133 women in two separate trials looked at whether aggressive early delivery via induction or cesarean section (interventionist management) was beneficial when compared with expectant management. One study was conducted in South Africa,[14] and one was conducted in the United States.[15] Both had 100% follow-up; both treated hypertension, and both gave betamethasone to the baby before delivery. The outcomes examined were renal failure rate, occurrence of HELLP syndrome, incidence of placental abruption, and death of the baby. For none of these outcome measures did interventionist or expectant management make a difference, despite the fact that delivery is the definitive cure for the disease.

FUTURE DIRECTIONS

Antiplatelet therapy for women at risk of developing preeclampsia is an intervention that demonstrates promise. A Cochrane review[16] comprising 59 trials and 37,650 women concluded that low-dose aspirin has moderate benefits including a 17% risk reduction in the development of preeclampsia. Antiplatelet agents also were associated with an 8% reduction in the relative risk of preterm births, and a 14% risk

---

Box 1
Suggested indications for delivery in preeclampsia and eclampsia

Fetal

    Age >38 weeks (term fetus)

    Severe fetal growth restriction

    Suspected fetal abruption

    Oligohydramnios

    Fetal distress

Maternal

    Thrombocytopenia with platelet count <100,000 cells/mm^3

    Worsening hepatic function

    Worsening renal insufficiency

    Severe persistent headache, visual changes

    Severe persistent epigastric pain and nausea, vomiting

Data from Schmidt D, Beck-Mannagetta G, Janz D, et al. The effect of pregnancy on the course of epilepsy: a prospective study. In: Janz D, Dam M, Richens A, et al, editors. Epilepsy, pregnancy, and the child. New York: Raven Press; 1982. p. 39–49.

---

reduction in fetal/neonatal death. Future directions should focus on deciphering which women are most likely to benefit, what dose should be used, and when the therapy should begin.

Other interventions studied for the prevention of preeclampsia and its complications include antioxidants,[17] Chinese herbal medicines,[18] nitric oxide donors,[19] progesterones,[20] bedrest,[21] exercise,[22] garlic,[23] and decreased salt consumption.[24] Systematic reviews of these studies report insufficient evidence to make any recommendations at this time.

SUMMARY

Eclampsia is a life-threatening emergency of which every emergency department physician should be aware. Immediate treatment is with magnesium sulfate 4 g intravenous bolus. This etiology of seizures should be suspected in all women of childbearing age.

KEY CONCEPTS

- Administer high-flow oxygen to all seizing pregnant patient to prevent fetal hypoxia. Twenty-five percent of eclamptic seizures occur in the postpartum period. Magnesium is the treatment of choice for eclamptic seizures.
- Labetalol and hydralazine are the antihypertensive agents of choice in eclampsia.
- The definitive treatment of eclampsia is delivery of the fetus.

REFERENCES

1. Holmes LB, Harvey EA, Coull BA, et al. The teratogenicity of anticonvulsant drugs. N Engl J Med 2001;344(15):1132–8.

2. Tatum WO. Balancing the risks to the fetus from epileptic seizures and antiepileptic drug exposure in pregnancy. Expert Rev Neurother 2009;9(12):1707–8.

3. ACOG educational bulletin. Seizure disorders in pregnancy. Number 231, December 1996. Committee on educational bulletins of the American college of obstetricians and gynecologists. Int J Gynaecol Obstet 1997;56(3):279–86.

4. Yerby MS, Friel PN, McCormick K, et al. Pharmacokinetics of anticonvulsants in pregnancy: alterations in plasma protein binding. Epilepsy Res 1990;5(3):223–8.

5. Schmidt D, Beck-Mannagetta G, Janz D, et al. The effect of pregnancy on the course of epilepsy: a prospective study. In: Janz D, Dam M, Richens A, et al, editors. Epilepsy, pregnancy, and the child. New York: Raven Press; 1982. p. 39–49.

6. Vajda FJ, Hitchcock A, Graham J, et al. Seizure control in antiepileptic drug-treated pregnancy. Epilepsia 2008;49(1):172–6.

7. Geographic variation in the incidence of hypertension in pregnancy. World Health Organization international collaborative study of hypertensive disorders of pregnancy. Am J Obstet Gynecol 1988;158(1):80–3.

8. Duley L, Henderson-Smart D. Magnesium sulphate versus phenytoin for eclampsia. Cochrane Database Syst Rev 2003;4:CD000128.

9. Duley L, Gulmezoglu AM, Henderson-Smart DJ. Magnesium sulphate and other anticonvulsants for women with preeclampsia. Cochrane Database Syst Rev 2003;2:CD000025.

10. Report of the national high blood pressure education program working group on high blood pressure in pregnancy. Am J Obstet Gynecol 2000;183(1):S1–22.

11. Duley L, Henderson-Smart D. Drugs for treatment of very high blood pressure during pregnancy. Cochrane Database Syst Rev 2006;3:CD001449.

12. Duley L, Williams J, Henderson-Smart D. Plasma volume expansion for treatment of pre-eclampsia. Cochrane Database Syst Rev 1999;4:CD001805. Updated 2010.

13. Churchiil D, Beevers GDC, Meher S, et al. Diuretics for preventing preeclampsia. Cochrane Database Syst Rev 2007;1:CD004451.

14. Odendaal HJ, Pattinson RC, Bam R, et al. Aggressive or expectant management for patients with severe preeclampsia between 28-34 weeks' gestation: a randomized controlled trial. Obstet Gynecol 1990;76(6):1070–5.

15. Sibai BM, Mercer BM, Schiff E, et al. Aggressive versus expectant management of severe preeclampsia at 28 to 32 weeks' gestation: a randomized controlled trial. Am J Obstet Gynecol 1994;171(3):818–22.

16. Knight M, Duley L, Henderson-Smart D, et al. Antiplatelet agents for preventing and treating preeclampsia. Cochrane Database Syst Rev 2007;2:CD004659.

17. Rubold A, Duley L, Crowther CA, et al. Antioxidants for preventing and treating pre-eclampsia. Cochrane Database Syst Rev 2008;1:CD004227.

18. Li W, Tang L, Wu T, et al. Chinese herbal medicines for treating pre-eclampsia. Cochrane Database Syst Rev 2006;2:CD005126.

19. Meher S, Duley L. Nitric oxide for preventing pre-eclampsia and its complications. Cochrane Database Syst Rev 2007;2:CD006490.

20. Meher S, Duley L. Progesterone for preventing preeclampsia and its complications. Cochrane Database Syst Rev 2006;4:CD006175.

21. Meher S, Duley L. Rest during pregnancy for preventing preeclampsia and its complications in women with normal blood pressure. Cochrane Database Syst Rev 2006;2:CD005939.

22. Meher S, Duley L. Exercise or other physical activity for preventing preeclampsia and its complications. Cochrane Database Syst Rev 2006;2:CD005942.

23. Meher S, Duley L. Garlic for preventing pre-eclampsia and its complications. Cochrane Database Syst Rev 2006;3:CD006065.

24. Duley L, Henderson-Smart DJ, Meher S. Altered dietary salt for preventing preeclampsia, and its complications. Cochrane Database Syst Rev 2005;4: CD005548.

Alcohol-Related Seizures

David McMicken, MD*, Jonathan L. Liss, MD

KEYWORDS

• Seizures • Alcohol withdrawal • Benzodiazepines

Among the various medical problems related to alcohol abuse, the differential diagnosis and management of seizures remains the most challenging and controversial problem. Any patient arriving to the emergency department (ED) with seizures should be questioned about alcohol intake. From 20% to 40% of patients with seizures who present to an ED have seizures related to alcohol abuse.[1] Alcohol is a causative factor in 15% to 24% of patients with status epilepticus.[2] The primary consideration in the initial care of these patients is the recognition and treatment of life-threatening causes of seizures, such as central nervous system (CNS) infection, hypoglycemia, and intracranial hematoma.

Alcohol may act in one of the several ways to produce seizures in patients with or without underlying foci:

- By partial or absolute withdrawal of alcohol after a period of chronic intake.
- By an acute alcohol-related metabolic brain disorder (eg, hypoglycemia, hyponatremia).
- By creating a situation leading to cerebral trauma.
- By precipitating seizures in patients with idiopathic or posttraumatic epilepsy.
- Persistent heavy intake of alcohol, independent of alcohol withdrawal.

Moreover, alcoholic patients are more susceptible to other disorders associated with seizures, including cerebral infarction, neurosyphilis, AIDS, brain abscess, meningitis, cerebral trauma, and subarachnoid hemorrhage (**Box 1**).[3–5]

ALCOHOL WITHDRAWAL SEIZURES

Chronic alcohol consumption affects central α-adrenergic and β-adrenergic receptors, the inhibitory neurotransmitter γ-aminobutyric acid, and dopamine turnover. The hallmark of alcohol withdrawal is CNS excitation with increased levels of cerebrospinal fluid (CSF) and plasma and urinary catecholamine.[6,7] The withdrawal syndrome develops 6 to 24 hours after the reduction of ethanol intake and usually

Department of Emergency Services, The Medical Center, Columbus, GA, USA
* Corresponding author.
E-mail address: David.McMicken@crhs.net

Emerg Med Clin N Am 29 (2011) 117–124
doi:10.1016/j.emc.2010.08.010
0733-8627/11/$ – see front matter © 2011 Elsevier Inc. All rights reserved.

Box 1
Differential diagnosis of alcohol-related seizures

Withdrawal (alcohol or drugs)

Exacerbation of an underlying seizure disorder

Acute drug intoxication (eg, amphetamines, anticholinergics, cocaine, isoniazid, organophosphates, tricyclics, salicylates)

Metabolic disorders (eg, hypoglycemia, hyponatremia, hypernatremia, hypocalcemia)

Infections (CNS or systemic)

Trauma (acute or remote)

Stroke

Noncompliance with anticonvulsants

---

lasts for 2 to 7 days. The alcohol withdrawal state ranges from mild withdrawal with insomnia and irritability to major withdrawal with diaphoresis, fever, disorientation, and hallucinations.[8]

Minor alcohol withdrawal syndrome occurs as early as 6 hours and usually peaks at 24 to 36 hours after the cessation or significant decrease in alcohol intake. It is characterized by mild autonomic hyperactivity including nausea, anorexia, tremor, tachycardia, hypertension, hyperreflexia, sleep disturbances (eg, insomnia, vivid dreams), and anxiety.[9] Major alcohol withdrawal syndrome occurs after more than 24 hours and usually peaks at 50 hours but occasionally takes up to 5 days after the decline or termination of drinking. This syndrome is characterized by anxiety that is more pronounced, insomnia, irritability, tremor, anorexia, tachycardia, hyperreflexia, hypertension, fever, decreased seizure threshold, auditory and visual hallucinations, and finally, delirium.[8–10]

Delirium tremens is at the extreme end of the alcohol withdrawal spectrum and is characterized by gross tremor, profound confusion, fever, incontinence, frightening visual hallucinations, and mydriasis. It seldom occurs before the third postabstinence day. Only 5% of patients hospitalized for alcohol withdrawal develop delirium tremens. True delirium tremens is rare and is not synonymous with alcohol withdrawal. Alcohol withdrawal seizures (AWS) can occur in minor alcohol withdrawal, major alcohol withdrawal, or delirium tremens.[9,10]

Alcohol withdrawal is one of the most common causes of adult-onset seizures. Descriptions of AWS were based on data collected by Victor and Brausch[11] on 241 alcohol abusers with seizures or alcohol-related illness complicated by seizures. These patients with AWS were confirmed to be alcoholic for many years, with the onset of seizures in adulthood. The seizures occurred 6 to 48 hours after the cessation of drinking. About 90% of the patients had 1 to 6 generalized tonic-clonic seizures, which occurred without warning, whereas 60% experienced multiple seizures, usually 2 to 4 within a 6-hour period. However, recent data suggest a much lower repeat seizure rate of 13% to 24%.[12] The incidence of partial (focal) seizures, common with posttraumatic epilepsy, is increased by alcohol withdrawal. However, partial seizures indicate a mass lesion until proven otherwise.

The term AWS is reserved for seizures with the characteristics described by Victor and Brausch.[11] The term alcohol-related seizures (ARS) is used to refer to all seizures in the aggregate associated with alcohol use, including the subset of AWS.

PATIENTS PRESENTING WITH A NORMAL NEUROLOGIC EXAMINATION
New-Onset ARS

Patients with new-onset ARS must be thoroughly evaluated, including alcoholic patients who claim to have had seizures in the past but for whom no documentation of previous seizures or of an appropriate workup is available. Possibility of metabolic disorders, toxin ingestion, infection, and structural abnormalities is ruled out by history, physical examination, and laboratory testing, including the estimation of levels of electrolytes, serum urea nitrogen, creatinine, glucose and computed tomographic (CT) scan, as necessary. An electroencephalography scheduled during follow-up may be considered (but its value is limited) in the patient with unexplained seizures.[13]

If the results of initial physical examination and laboratory tests are normal, patients who remain seizure free and symptom free with no sign of withdrawal after 4 to 6 hours of observation may be discharged. Optimal outpatient treatment include clear guidelines for follow-up and reevaluation and the help of a concerned family member or friend (who is not a drinking partner) who should remain with the patient for 1 to 2 days. These criteria may be difficult to meet, and the physician must use discretion in deciding to admit for observation when the patient is at risk of serious injury. The ideal disposition is participation in a detoxification/rehabilitation program.

It may be unclear whether the patient has had AWS or the new onset of a seizure disorder in the setting of alcohol consumption. At this point, such a patient probably does not require further treatment. The literature provides little information about the natural history, including the risk of subsequent seizures, in patients in the ED, presenting with an unprovoked seizure. Beginning anticonvulsant treatment in a patient after a new-onset single seizure is controversial, and the final decision regarding treatment should be individualized and made after consultation with a neurologist or the patient's primary care provider. The patient with first-time ARS, who has a history that is consistent with AWS and a workup with negative results can be treated as presented in the following sections.[14]

Alert patients with a history of prior seizures, during alcohol withdrawal

Alcoholic patients with the manifestations of alcohol withdrawal, who have not had a recent seizure but have a related history of AWS are encountered frequently in the ED. The risk of seizure increases 10-fold in this subset of patients.[15,16]

Benzodiazepines alone are sufficient to prevent AWS.[12] Many of patients with AWS sporadically take one or more anticonvulsants. It is difficult, if not impossible, to determine in the ED whether these anticonvulsants were given for an underlying seizure disorder or AWS. To effectively prevent AWS, detoxification with benzodiazepines should be initiated early, because most AWS occur within the first 24 hours after alcohol withdrawal. Treatment should be started with the understanding that the patient will be observed for 4 to 6 hours and referred to a detoxification/rehabilitation program (if available).

An initial test dose of 2 mg of lorazepam or 10 mg of diazepam can be given orally or 1 mg of lorazepam or 5 mg of diazepam intravenously to the patient in the ED. This dose may be repeated depending on the patient's response. The patient is observed for 4 to 6 hours, which guides the dose required for outpatient treatment. Prescribing anticonvulsants, such as benzodiazepines (other than a short 3- to 6-day course for alcohol withdrawal) and phenytoin, to the discharged alcoholic patient may increase the potential for addiction or may paradoxically increase the number of acute seizures. For a concurrent seizure disorder, the poorly compliant alcoholic patient may do better without anticonvulsants prescribed for outpatients.[15] Therefore, the ideal disposition is admission to a detoxification/rehabilitation unit.

Alert patients with a seizure, before or after presentation

Alcoholic patients with a documented history of ARS, who experience a single seizure or a short burst of seizures should be treated with lorazepam, 2 mg intravenously. These patients usually require observation with careful monitoring of neurologic status for at least 6 hours, before discharge.[12]

PATIENTS WITH AN ABNORMAL NEUROLOGIC PRESENTATION
New-Onset Partial Seizure

Partial (focal) seizures are reported to account for up to 24% of ARS. Conversely, studies have shown that 17% to 21% of patients with partial ARS have structural lesions (hematomas, tumors, or vascular abnormalities).[17] These primary causes of partial ARS, such as prior head trauma, may be missed in the history taking. As a result, an emergent CT scan is indicated to evaluate new-onset partial seizures.

The patient with a documented history of focal ARS, who has been previously evaluated does not require an emergency CT scan, provided a return to baseline occurs promptly. A patient presenting with focal ARS with subsequent normal neurologic imaging can be managed with supportive care, observation for 6 hours, and treatment with benzodiazepine for withdrawal signs or symptoms. Appropriate follow-up should be arranged.

MANAGEMENT

Historically, up to one-third of patients with AWS progressed to delirium tremens because of inadequate treatment. Currently, this proportion has decreased to less than 5% with early aggressive benzodiazepine therapy.[18]

An intravenous line of normal saline should be established. If the patient has an altered mental status, administration of thiamine, magnesium, dextrose, and naloxone should be considered. Empirical glucose bolus dosing should not be prescribed if a prompt and accurate determination of blood glucose levels is possible.[19]

Although magnesium does not decrease the severity of withdrawal symptoms or the incidence of delirium or seizures, it carries no significant risk or cost. In the nonacute setting, oral magnesium supplementation in long-term alcoholic patients improves liver function test results, electrolyte balance, and muscle strength.[20] Intravenous administration of multivitamin preparations may be considered for chronic malnutrition but their clinical benefit is not proven.

Obtundation

The obtunded or stuporous alcohol-dependent patient with a history of seizure poses a diagnostic challenge. The patient's decreased level of consciousness (LOC) may be because of a postictal state, an occult head trauma, an unrecognized metabolic disorder, or poisoning. The first task is to determine the possibility of hypoglycemia (diagnosed and reversed at the bedside in seconds to minutes) or a neurosurgical lesion with morbidity and mortality directly related to the time of surgical intervention.

Patients with focal neurologic findings on physical examination, new-onset seizures, partial (focal) seizures, or evidence of acute head trauma should be considered for an urgent CT scan. If the LOC is consistently improving, the patient is unlikely to have an immediate life-threatening problem. An unimproved or deteriorating LOC requires an urgent CT scan.

No History of Seizure/No Current Seizure

In the patient with alcohol withdrawal who lacks a history of seizures, benzodiazepines generally have sufficient anticonvulsant activity to prevent withdrawal seizures.[21]

Status Epilepticus

Although fewer than 8% of patients with ARS progress to status epilepticus, alcohol is implicated in 15% to 24% of patients with status epilepticus.[22] Status epilepticus may also be the first presentation of ARS. The most common cause of status epilepticus is discontinuation of or erratic compliance with an anticonvulsant drug regimen, followed by ARS. However, status epilepticus may occur for a variety of reasons and is often multifactorial. Thus, it is essential to screen for all possible factors underlying repeated or prolonged seizures, even when a probable cause is thought to be readily apparent.

Initial interventions for the alcoholic in status epilepticus include stabilization of the airway, breathing, and circulation; administration of glucose and thiamine as indicated; and treatment with a benzodiazepine. Lorazepam and diazepam are both effective in terminating seizures in status epilepticus. Lorazepam is preferable because its anticonvulsant effect lasts several hours, whereas diazepam's anticonvulsant effect lasts only from 20 to 30 minutes. Because of this short-term effect lorazepam has fewer recurrent seizures and requires fewer repeat doses than diazepam.[23–25]

If seizures persist after lorazepam or diazepam administration, a loading dose of phenytoin, 20 mg/kg, or fosphenytoin, 15 to 20 phenytoin equivalent mg/kg, is administered in the second intravenous line. Additional doses of 5 mg/kg of phenytoin, to a maximum of 30 mg/kg, can be given if status is not terminated.[23]

Most of the cardiac abnormalities associated with phenytoin infusion are caused by its solvent propylene glycol. Caution is advised in patients who have preexisting heart disease. Using a 20-gauge intravenous line proximal to the forearm to avoid purple glove syndrome and keeping the phenytoin rate less than 50 mg/min can minimize the problem of hypotension and bradycardia. Fosphenytoin does not contain propylene glycol and is safe and well tolerated at intravenous rates of 100 to 150 mg/min.

Rapid achievement of therapeutic free phenytoin levels, without significant side effects, has been documented using fosphenytoin in patients with status epilepticus.[26] However, the benefit of fosphenytoin versus phenytoin in the ED has been questioned.[26–30]

Phenobarbital was recommended in the past for patients who fail to respond to benzodiazepine and phenytoin. Experts have suggested skipping phenobarbital for refractory status and initiating infusion of pentobarbital, propofol, or midazolam.[23,31–35]

It is often difficult to rule out a CNS infection in alcoholic patients with status epilepticus because of concomitant hyperthermia, serum leukocytosis, and CSF pleocytosis. If CSF infection is a possibility, intravenous antibiotic therapy should be started, blood cultures obtained, and a lumbar puncture considered.[36]

PHENYTOIN/ANTICONVULSANT CONUNDRUM

Phenytoin has no significant benefit over placebo in preventing recurrence of AWS.[1,37] Considering the risks of phenytoin and no demonstrated benefit in the setting of AWS, it is not indicated for the treatment of AWS. The sudden withdrawal of phenytoin administration may induce the convulsive effects of alcohol withdrawal. Withdrawal seizures may occur in epileptic patients withdrawn from phenytoin treatment. In patients with status epilepticus, alcohol and noncompliance with anticonvulsant regimens may be synergistic.[20,38]

Alcoholic patients with preexisting seizure disorders pose a dilemma when they are supposed to be taking antiepileptic drugs (AEDs) but their blood levels suggest noncompliance. This situation is especially problematic when their epileptic attacks are uncommon and seem to occur exclusively in the context of alcohol withdrawal. Some of these patients may have AWS and may have been misdiagnosed. Others may have a seizure disorder that seems to be confined to the setting of alcohol withdrawal. Such patients have demonstrated that they cannot maintain compliance with their treatment.

A patient taking an AED for an antecedent seizure disorder, which presents with a seizure while intoxicated, falls into a different category. Such an episode could be an isolated event in a usually compliant patient without a history of chronic alcohol abuse. In this patient, a seizure in the setting of a subtherapeutic AED level may represent the consequences of noncompliance with the AED versus AWS.[39]

FUTURE DIRECTIONS

In this age of computerized medicine, it will soon be possible to have a complete medical history on even the most obtunded ED patient. This advancement will go a long way in helping the emergency physician determine if the alcohol-related seizure is an isolated event or a recurrent problem. It will help determine if the patient an epileptic whose presentation is complicated by alcohol or if alcohol is the sole problem. This kind of comprehensive history should help reduce the cost of emergency medicine care by reducing the number of imaging studies and other tests that are currently deemed necessary.

Moreover, as researchers continue to evaluate genetic markers, which may demonstrate a predisposition to ARS, and easily measured biomarkers, such as serum prolactin and homocysteine levels, it may one day be possible to accurately predict which patients are at risk for withdrawal seizures. Therefore, it may one day be possible to accurately separate patients in need of prophylaxis from those in whom seizure treatment is unnecessary.

SUMMARY

Alcohol kills the person who consumes it and it kills unintended victims by the acts of inebriated persons. Whatever medical, traumatic, psychological, or social problem brings an alcoholic patient to the ED, the underlying problem is alcoholism and the ultimate goal is abstinence. Most municipalities have either an Alcoholics Anonymous chapter or a treatment center for anyone who desires help with alcohol. In small communities, clergy or social workers can usually arrange rehabilitation programs. This disease will surely progress if alcoholism is not recognized and the patient is not given the opportunity to participate in a rehabilitation program. It is up to the emergency physician to intervene on behalf of the patient and the public.[40,41]

KEY CONCEPTS

- Not all ARS are AWS
- Search for reversible causes (eg, hypoglycemia, intracranial hemorrhage, CNS infection) in alcoholic patients with seizures
- Obtain a CT scan of the head in alcoholic patients with a seizure of undetermined cause
- Lorazepam is the drug of choice in alcoholic patients who have had a seizure or who are demonstrating signs of withdrawal
- Alcoholic patients who have had a seizure should generally be observed for 4 to 6 hours and, if discharged, referred to a detoxificaton/rehabilitation program, if possible

ACKNOWLEDGMENTS

The authors wish to thank Alisha Miles and Laurie Hodgen for their research on this project.

REFERENCES

1. Rathlev NK, D'Onofrio G, Fish SS, et al. The lack of efficacy of phenytoin in the prevention of recurrent alcohol-related seizures. Ann Emerg Med 1994;23(3):513–8.
2. Lowenstein DH, Alldredge BK. Status epilepticus at an urban public hospital in the 1980s. Neurology 1993;43(3 Pt 1):483–8.
3. Brust JC. Acute neurologic complications of drug and alcohol abuse. Neurol Clin 1998;16(2):503–19.
4. Lacy JR, Filley CM, Earnest MP, et al. Brain infarction and hemorrhage in young and middle-aged adults. West J Med 1984;141(3):329–34.
5. Ng SK, Hauser WA, Brust JC, et al. Alcohol consumption and withdrawal in new-onset seizures. N Engl J Med 1988;319:666–73.
6. Rosenbloom A. Emerging treatment options in the alcohol withdrawal syndrome. J Clin Psychiatry 1988;49(Suppl):28–32.
7. Coomes TR, Smith SW. Successful use of propofol in refractory delirium tremens. Ann Emerg Med 1997;30(6):825–8.
8. Isbell H, Fraser HF, Wikler A, et al. An experimental study of the etiology of rum fits and delirium tremens. Q J Stud Alcohol 1955;16(1):1–33.
9. Turner RC, Lichstein PR, Peden JG Jr, et al. Alcohol withdrawal syndromes: a review of pathophysiology, clinical presentation, and treatment. J Gen Intern Med 1989;4(5):432–44.
10. Adinoff B, Bone GH, Linnoila M. Acute ethanol poisoning and the ethanol withdrawal syndrome. Med Toxicol Adverse Drug Exp 1988;3(3):172–96.
11. Victor M, Brausch C. The role of abstinence in the genesis of alcoholic epilepsy. Epilepsia 1967;8(1):1–20.
12. D'Onofrio G, Rathlev NK, Ulrich AS, et al. Lorazepam for the prevention of recurrent seizures related to alcohol. N Engl J Med 1999;340(12):915–9.
13. Sand T, Brathen G, Michler R, et al. Clinical utility of EEG in alcohol-related seizures. Acta Neurol Scand 2002;105(1):18–24.
14. Scheuer ML, Pedley TA. The evaluation and treatment of seizures. N Engl J Med 1990;323(21):1468–74.
15. Hillbom ME, Hjelm-Jäger M. Should alcohol withdrawal seizures be treated with anti-epileptic drugs? Acta Neurol Scand 1984;69(1):39–42.
16. Marx J, Berner J, Bar-Or D, et al. Prophylaxis of alcohol withdrawal seizures: a prospective study [abstract]. Ann Emerg Med 1986;15:637.
17. Earnest MP, Feldman H, Marx JA, et al. Intracranial lesions shown by CT scans in 259 cases of first alcohol-related seizures. Neurology 1988;38(10):1561–5.
18. Koch-Weser J, Sellers EM, Kalant H. Alcohol intoxication and withdrawal. N Engl J Med 1976;294(14):757–62.
19. Sieber FE, Traystman RJ. Special issues: glucose and the brain. Crit Care Med 1992;20(1):104–14.
20. Gullestad L, Dolva LO, Soyland E, et al. Oral magnesium supplementation improves metabolic variables and muscle strength in alcoholics. Alcohol Clin Exp Res 1992;16(5):986–90.
21. Haddox VG, Bidder TG, Waldron LE, et al. Clorazepate use may prevent alcohol withdrawal convulsions. West J Med 1987;146(6):695–6.

22. Lowenstein DH. Status epilepticus: an overview of the clinical problem. Epilepsia 1999;40(Suppl 1):S3–8 [discussion: S21–2].
23. Treatment of convulsive status epilepticus. Recommendations of the Epilepsy Foundation of America's Working Group on Status Epilepticus. JAMA 1993;270(7):854–9.
24. Cock HR, Schapira AH. A comparison of lorazepam and diazepam as initial therapy in convulsive status epilepticus. QJM 2002;95(4):225–31.
25. Alldredge BK, Gelb AM, Isaacs SM, et al. A comparison of lorazepam, diazepam, and placebo for the treatment of out-of-hospital status epilepticus. N Engl J Med 2001;345(9):631–7.
26. Johnson J, Wrenn K. Inappropriate fosphenytoin use in the ED. Am J Emerg Med 2001;19(4):293–4.
27. Coplin WM, Rhoney DH, Rebuck JA, et al. Randomized evaluation of adverse events and length-of-stay with routine emergency department use of phenytoin or fosphenytoin. Neurol Res 2002;24(8):842–8.
28. Touchette DR, Rhoney DH. Cost-minimization analysis of phenytoin and fosphenytoin in the emergency department. Pharmacotherapy 2000;20(8):908–16.
29. Rudis MI, Touchette DR, Swadron SP, et al. Cost-effectiveness of oral phenytoin, intravenous phenytoin, and intravenous fosphenytoin in the emergency department. Ann Emerg Med 2004;43(3):386–97.
30. Horowitz BZ. Fosphenytoin farewell? Ann Emerg Med 2004;43(3):398–400.
31. Shorvon S. The management of status epilepticus. J Neurol Neurosurg Psychiatr 2001;70(Suppl 2):II22–7.
32. Rosenow F, Arzimanoglou A, Baulac M. Recent developments in treatment of status epilepticus: a review. Epileptic Disord 2002;4(Suppl 2):S41–51.
33. Wheless JW. Acute management of seizures in the syndromes of idiopathic generalized epilepsies. Epilepsia 2003;44(Suppl 2):22–6.
34. Smith BJ. Treatment of status epilepticus. Neurol Clin 2001;19(2):347–69.
35. Yu KT, Mills S, Thompson N, et al. Safety and efficacy of intravenous valproate in pediatric status epilepticus and acute repetitive seizures. Epilepsia 2003;44(5):724–6.
36. Wrenn KD, Larson S. The febrile alcoholic in the emergency department. Am J Emerg Med 1991;9(1):57–60.
37. Chance JF. Emergency department treatment of alcohol withdrawal seizures with phenytoin. Ann Emerg Med 1991;20(5):520–2.
38. Sellers EM. Alcohol, barbiturate and benzodiazepine withdrawal syndromes: clinical management. CMAJ 1988;139(2):113–20.
39. Simon RP. Alcohol and seizures. N Engl J Med 1988;319(11):715–6.
40. Davidson P, Koziol-McLain J, Harrison L, et al. Intoxicated ED patients: a 5-year follow-up of morbidity and mortality. Ann Emerg Med 1997;30(5):593–7.
41. Ary RD, Wald MM, Rutland-Brown W. Alcohol still kills! Ann Emerg Med 2002;39(6):651–2.

Toxin-Related Seizures

Adhi N. Sharma, MD[a,b,*], Robert J. Hoffman, MD[c]

KEYWORDS

- Toxin-related seizures • NMDA receptor
- GABA receptor complex • Benzodiazepines

Toxin-related seizures are secondary to an imbalance in the brain's equilibrium of excitation-inhibition. This delicate balance is maintained via excitatory neurotransmission (eg, glutamate or the N-methyl-D-aspartate [NMDA] receptor) and inhibitory neurotransmission (eg, γ–aminobutyric acid [GABA] or the GABA receptor complex). Balance is also dependent on normal ion flux and homeostasis of biogenic amines and acetylcholine. Perturbation of this equilibrium can be the result of the presence of a toxin or the abrupt removal of one (withdrawal). This article reviews the epidemiology, pathophysiology, toxicology, clinical features, and management of toxin-related seizures. Particular emphasis is placed on contrasting the management of toxin-related seizures with seizures of other etiologies, because clinicians are likely to have greater experience, knowledge, and comfort dealing with the latter. Despite the differences, the basic management principles for any seizure are the same: rapidly stabilize the patient and provide supportive care; expediently terminate seizure activity; diagnose the cause of the seizure; and abate associated morbidity and mortality.

EPIDEMIOLOGY

The true incidence of toxin-related seizure is unknown. Prospective study of patients presenting with their first convulsive seizure has found the following: 8.5% of patients older than 25 years have a toxic/metabolic etiology[1]; 11% of patients older than 60 years have a toxic/metabolic etiology[2]; and 24% of patients between 40 and 65 years of age have a toxic/metabolic/vascular etiology.[3] Because there is no discrete reporting of toxin-induced seizures, these data only give parameters within

---

[a] Department of Emergency Medicine, Good Samaritan Hospital Medical Center, West Islip, NY 11795, USA
[b] Department of Emergency Medicine, Mount Sinai School of Medicine, One Gustave Levy Place, New York, NY 10029, USA
[c] Department of Emergency Medicine, Beth Israel Medical Center, 1st Avenue at 16th Street, New York, NY 10003, USA
* Corresponding author. Department of Emergency Medicine, Good Samaritan Hospital Medical Center, West Islip, NY 11795.
E-mail address: ansharma@pol.net

Emerg Med Clin N Am 29 (2011) 125–139
doi:10.1016/j.emc.2010.08.011
0733-8627/11/$ – see front matter © 2011 Elsevier Inc. All rights reserved.

which the incidence of toxin-related seizures might lie. Retrospective study of first seizure in patients older than 16 years has found 6% of new-onset seizures to be toxin related.[4] In a prospective study of human immunodeficiency virus–positive adults with first seizure, 47% were toxin related.[5]

Box 1 presents a list of the more common agents associated with seizures. Certain toxins impart an elevated risk for seizure[6]: 19%[7] to 87%[8] of isoniazid ingestions; 15%[9] to 37%[10] of buproprion ingestions, and 14% of venlafaxine ingestions.[11] Clinicians should also be cognizant of iatrogenic causes of toxin-related seizures related to the use of local anesthetic agents and flumazenil.[12–14]

PATHOPHYSIOLOGY

There are 4 mechanisms that are associated with toxin-induced seizures:

1. Activity at NMDA and GABA receptors, including GABA synthesis with resultant imbalance in excitation and inhibition
2. Disturbances of ion flux, usually involving sodium channels (either blockade or openers); this alters the resting potential of neural cells (either depolarization or hyperpolarization)
3. Adenosine antagonism
4. Alterations in concentration or activity of biogenic amines and acetylcholine. This mechanism is typified by the fact that seizures may result from either cholinergic excess or an anticholinergic state.

Though seemingly abstract, an understanding of the underlying mechanism can play a significant role in treatment. Despite the numerous mechanisms described, most toxins induce seizures via activity at the GABA receptor complex.

Glutamate/NMDA and GABA

Excitatory neural tone that leads to seizure is mediated predominantly by glutamate, aspartate, and similar excitatory neurotransmitters binding at NMDA receptors.[15–17] The counterbalancing inhibitory tone is mediated predominantly by GABA as well as endogenous benzodiazepine-like neurotransmitters at GABA receptors. Excessive excitatory amino acid (EAA) tone is associated with seizure,[18,19] while increasing GABA activity results in sedation and ultimately coma.[20,21] Consciousness is maintained by balancing excitation and inhibition.

Toxin-related seizures as a result of imbalance of EAA and GABA are usually the result of inhibition of GABA tone, which is effectively excitation. EAA concentrations may be increased directly by toxins such as cocaine, or indirectly by toxins that induce ischemia, hypoxia, or hypoglycemia.[22] In either instance, the net effect may result in seizure activity. Toxins that disrupt metabolism, such as hypoglycemic agents, cyanide,[23] and carbon monoxide, result in elevated EAA levels and may cause seizure.[24–26]

Drugs effecting glutamate/NMDA antagonism typically have potent anticonvulsant and neuroprotective effects whereas those effecting glutamate/NMDA agonism have proconvulsant effects.[27,28] Nearly all pharmaceutical agents with pure NMDA agonism or antagonism effects are experimental drugs. Imperfect examples of such agents include the anticonvulsant lamotrigine, which diminishes excessive EAA activity,[29] and toxins such as cocaine[30,31] or soman,[32] which work in part by increasing excitatory amino acids.

Box 1
Partial list of seizure-inducing toxins

Anticholinergics
    Diphenhydramine[a]
Anticonvulsants
    Carbamazepine[a]
    Phenytoin
Cholinergic agents
    Organophosphates
    Nerve agents
Hydrazines
    Isoniazid
Hydrocarbons
    Camphor
    Lindane
Hypoglycemic agents
    Insulin
    Sulfonylureas
Methylxanthines
    Theophylline[a]
    Caffeine
Miscellaneous
    Buproprion
    Citalopram
    Lithium
    Venlafaxine[a]
Mitochondrial Toxins
    Carbon monoxide
    Cyanide
Opioids
    Meperidine
    Propoxyphene[a]
Sodium Channel Blockers
    Lidocaine[a]
    Cyclic antidepressants[a]
Sympathomimetics
    Amphetamines
    Cocaine
Withdrawal
    Ethanol
    Sedative-hypnotic

[a] Toxins also associated with cardiotoxicity and dysrhythmias.

GABA agonists, for example, benzodiazepines or barbiturates, have anticonvulsant effects, whereas GABA antagonists such as flumazenil,[13] lindane,[33] or pentylenetetrazole (Metrazol) have proconvulsant effects.

Inadequate GABA Production

GABA is synthesized from glutamate via a pathway that uses glutamic acid decarboxylase (GAD). GAD requires pyridoxal 5′-phosphate as a cofactor (the active form of pyridoxine). Hydrazines such as isoniazid or *Gyrometra* sp mushrooms disrupt normal production of GABA by numerous mechanisms including blocking pyridoxal 5′-phosphate and enhancing the elimination of pydridoxine. The ultimate toxic effect of hydrazines is an inadequate quantity of GABA, which may result in seizures. In this unique circumstance, use of benzodiazepine or barbiturate anticonvulsants may be ineffective because both require GABA to exert their clinical effect, and in this setting central nervous system GABA concentrations are inadequate. Pyridoxine (vitamin B6) is critical in the management of seizures related to hydrazine poisoning, and is purported to be beneficial in theophylline toxicity,[34] which may depress pyridoxine levels through an unknown mechanism of action.[35]

Disruption of Normal Ionic Flux

Brain neurons are continuously dependent on appropriate ion flux to maintain a given state of polarization, depolarization, or repolarization. Seizures may result from an imbalance, and shifting of a given neurologic state out of homeostasis. Whether by increasing sodium channel blockade or sodium channel opening, or increasing either anticholinergic or cholinergic tone, deviation from homeostasis in either direction can result in seizure. **Box 2** provides examples of toxins that affect ion flux and are associated with seizures.[36]

Box 2
Toxins that induce seizure via ion flux and their related mechanisms

Sodium Channel Blockers

   Camphor

   Lidocaine

   Phenytoin

   Quinidine

Sodium Channel Openers

   Ciguatoxin

   Pyrethroids

Potassium Channel Blockers

   4-Aminopyridine

Potassium Channel Openers

   Barium

   Apamin (bee venom)

β-Adrenergic antagonists

   Propranolol

Adenosine Activity in Seizures

Adenosine is the endogenous neurotransmitter that is responsible for interictal periods. When a seizure does not self-terminate, both EAA levels and GABA levels increase[37] and adenosine release occurs in a burst fashion,[38] resulting in brief electrical silence followed by a resumption of nonictal brainwave activity (**Fig. 1**).[39] Any interference with this process may result in seizures without interictal periods, clinically evident as status epilepticus. Methylxanthines, such as caffeine and theophylline, are structural analogues of adenosine that do not possess any activity at the adenosine receptor and therefore act as adenosine antagonists. Accordingly, theophylline toxicity is often marked by refractory seizures (see **Fig. 1**). Caffeine and theophylline have been used to induce more robust and prolonged seizure activity in patients undergoing electroconvulsive therapy.[40–42] A familiar analogy to this activity is therapeutic use of adenosine to treat tachydysrhythmias. Administration typically results in brief electrical silence (asystole) followed by resumption of normal electrical activity. Adenosine has been reported to have significant efficacy as an anticonvulsant in toxin-related seizures, though further research is needed before it can be recommended as a therapeutic modality.[43,44]

The dangers of toxic doses of adenosine antagonists in the setting of toxin-related seizures are well known: Status epilepticus associated with theophylline has as high as a 23% incidence of death and a 50% incidence of death or permanent neurologic disability.[45] Seizure activity in a patient with theophylline or caffeine poisoning that is unresponsive to benzodiazepine therapy is also unlikely to respond to phenytoin administration, but may respond well to barbiturate therapy.[46,47]

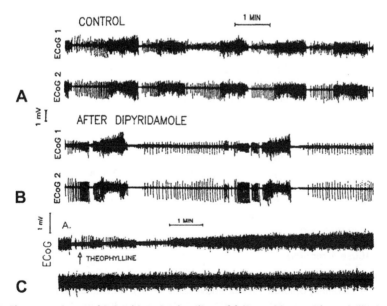

Fig. 1. Electrocorticographic ictal-interictal cycling of feline subjects with penicillin-induced seizures. (A) Control. (B) Prolonged interictal phase after dipyridamole (adenosine reuptake inhibitor). (C) Status epilepticus after theophylline administration. (*Reproduced from* Eldridge FL, Paydarfar D, Scott SC, et al. Role of endogenous adenosine in recurrent generalized seizures. Exp Neurol 1989;103(2):179–85; with permission.)

There are numerous toxins capable of causing seizure that do not fit neatly into the aforementioned categories. Other toxins, such as cocaine, which both increases glutamate release but also acts as a sodium channel blocker, may have multiple mechanisms that induce seizures. Fortunately, the fundamental treatment strategy for toxin-related seizures can be broadly applied, as it is independent of the mechanism by which the seizure was induced.

COMPLICATIONS ASSOCIATED WITH TOXIN-RELATED SEIZURES

Complications associated with toxin-related seizures carry significant risks of morbidity and sometimes mortality. Although most toxin-related seizures are not fatal, if status epilepticus is induced the chance of mortality is increased. Toxin-related seizures can result in serious cardiovascular effects. Seizure in an otherwise toxic but stable patient may precipitate dysrhythmias or cardiac arrest, particularly for drugs that affect cardiac conduction or rhythm (see **Box 1**).[11,48–56]

Aberrant cardiac conduction, specifically prolonged QRS duration, predicts the likelihood of seizure and occurs with seizure in patients with cyclic antidepressant overdose.[57] This phenomenon of cardiac conduction abnormality associated with seizure appears to occur with other seizure-inducing toxins that also affect cardiac conduction, but not with seizures resulting from epilepsy.[58] However, seizure with other agents, such as antidysrhythmics, may occur in the absence of an electrocardiograph (ECG) abnormality.[59]

INVESTIGATIONS

Bedside assessment of serum glucose and 12-lead ECG should be used routinely in the evaluation of patients with undifferentiated seizures. Other investigations are discussed here, but are not routinely indicated for toxin-related seizures.

Computed Tomography

Computed tomography (CT) should be selectively used for patients with toxin-related seizures. One study did not find any benefit to routine brain CT performed on all patients presenting with altered mental status associated with poisoning or drug overdose.[60] However, in a large study of patients presenting with a first alcohol-related seizure, 6.2% of patients had intracranial lesions discovered by CT.[61] These varying data are the result of the spectrum of problems that result in toxin-related seizures.

In patients with poisoning that reasonably would be presumed to cause seizure but who have no focal neurologic deficit, a head CT scan is not necessary in the emergency department. This situation requires determination that the seizure is expected to result from the toxin or withdrawal and correlation of the patient's clinical presentation, to determine that the toxin exposure or withdrawal in question is a likely cause of the seizure in question.

Drug of Abuse Screening

Of the drugs of abuse commonly screened for, namely amphetamines, cannabinoids (marijuana), cocaine, opioids, and phencyclidine (PCP), only cocaine is a regular and reliable cause of seizure. In the absence of overt cocaine toxicity, seizure associated with cocaine exposure should not be attributed to this drug. Synthetic opioids (eg, meperidine and propoxyphene) associated with seizure are not detected by routine opioid screening assays. Amphetamines other than 3,4-methylenedioxymethamphetamine (MDMA; "Ecstasy") as well as PCP infrequently cause seizures. PCP and amphetamines other than MDMA are only anecdotally associated with seizure[62] and actually have anticonvulsant properties at most sublethal doses.[63–66]

Other than cocaine, it is highly unlikely that a drug of abuse responsible for a seizure would be detected with routine drug of abuse screening. Cocaine-induced seizures occur in only a minority of cocaine users and therefore should be evaluated in the same manner as any first seizure. As such, in the opinion of the authors, drug of abuse screening with the intent of using the results to diagnose or medically manage patients with toxin-related seizures has no clinical value and is not recommended.

Electroencephalograph Monitoring

Electroencephalograph (EEG) monitoring is indicated for all patients who have been paralyzed, for the purpose of supportive care during seizure activity. Neuromuscular blockade can facilitate endotracheal intubation for control of airway, and subsequent oxygenation and ventilation and temperature regulation is improved when heat-generating motor activity ceases. However, despite the absence of motor activity, status epilepticus in the paralyzed patient imparts a significant risk of permanent neurologic injury or even death.[67] Whenever possible, EEG monitoring should be performed in the paralyzed patient to ensure appropriate anticonvulsive therapy. The pupillary light response has been demonstrated to be preserved during neuromuscular blockade and barbiturate coma, and may be used as a surrogate when continuous EEG monitoring is unavailable.[68] During generalized seizure activity, pupils are typically dilated secondary to the associated catecholamine surge, effectively extinguishing pupillary response to light. Nonetheless, clinicians should be hesitant to initiate prolonged paralysis in the patient with status epilepticus if EEG monitoring is not available.

Several toxins, such as strychnine, tetanus toxin, and γ-hydroxybutyrate, as well as circumstances such as serotonin syndrome, may result in myoclonus, tremor, tetany, or other motor activity that may be difficult to distinguish from seizure activity. If there is any question about the presence of seizure activity, an EEG is indicated.

MANAGEMENT OF TOXIN-RELATED SEIZURES

Supportive care is the most important aspect of toxin-related seizure management. Airway management with appropriate oxygenation and ventilation in conjunction with blood pressure, heart rate, and core temperature stabilization are critical areas of support. In addition, attention must be paid to maintaining appropriate serum glucose and pH. Unfortunately, despite optimal supportive care, permanent neurologic sequela is possible from uncontrolled seizure activity.

Although seizure activity is often self-limited, at times specific anticonvulsant therapies are necessary. Therapeutic regimens designed for epileptic seizures applied to toxin-related seizures can be effective or potentially harmful. As such, the authors recommend an algorithm for managing toxin-related seizures, which is safe if applied to epileptic seizures as well (**Fig. 2**). Terminating toxin-related seizures is not effected by a simple strategy to restore "balance." For example, sodium channel blockade–induced seizure is not treated with sodium channel openers: Treatment does not consist of treating with the "equal and opposite" therapeutic agent, but rather by effecting neural sedation by means of supportive care and, in most cases, administration of medications to increase GABA tone.

Initial management of any seizure is identical regardless of the seizure etiology. After airway and cardiopulmonary issues have been addressed and an assessment of

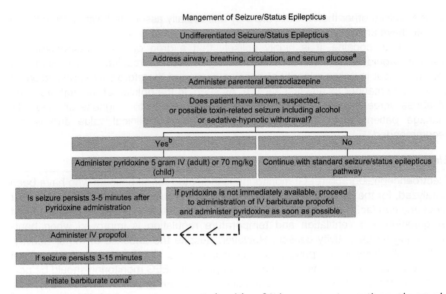

Fig. 2. Toxin-related seizure management algorithm. [a] It is necessary to continuously reevaluate and correct airway, breathing, circulation, serum glucose, electrolyte, temperature and vital signs abnormalities as appropriate. [b] If diagnosis of specific poisoning is made or suspected, a specific antidote, such as the cyanide antidote kit, physostigmine, atropine, or pralidoxime, may be indicated. [c] Rapid-acting barbiturates such as pentobarbital or thiopental preferred, phenobarbital is acceptable. Rapid-acting barbiturates are expected to work within 3 to 5 minutes; the therapeutic effect of phenobarbital may take 15 minutes or longer.

serum glucose has been made, administration of a benzodiazepine is indicated. If, within several minutes, the seizure activity does not terminate, an additional dose of benzodiazepine should be administered. Although the seizure termination efficacy of diazepam, lorazepam, and midazolam appear to be similar, lorazepam has benefits with regard to longer duration of activity,[69] and midazolam is the best choice for intramuscular administration.[70]

Benzodiazepines

Benzodiazepines remain the mainstay of seizure therapy. While there is often discussion related to which benzodiazepine should be given first, there should be no delay in administering any benzodiazepine to the patient in status epilepticus. Lorazepam is the preferred initial benzodiazepine and can be given to adults at 2 mg/min up to 4 mg and repeated once at 10 minutes if needed. Pediatric (1 month to 12 years) dosing is: 0.05–0.1 mg/kg (maximum: 4 mg/dose) slow IV over 2-5 minutes (maximum rate: 2 mg/minute); may repeat every 10–15 minutes if needed. Diazepam dosing is 5–10 mg IV in adults repeated every 10 minutes as needed to a maximum of 30 mg. Pediatric (1 month to 5 years) dosing is 0.2-0.5 mg/kg IV to a maximum dose of 5 mg, children over 5 years old can receive 1 mg every 2-5 minutes as needed to a maximum of 10 mg. Midazolam has been shown to be effective even when administered via non-intravenous routes. The adult IV dosing for midazolam in status epilepticus is 1–2.5 mg in 2 minute intervals to a maximum of 10 mg. Pediatric dosing is 0.05–0.1 mg/kg to a maximum of dose of 6 mg. Midazolam should be given slowly as it can cause cardiac arrest and has an FDA black box warning to this effect. Also of note, high dose midazolam has been shown to terminate seizure activity refractory to other agents and may be considered as a life-saving measure.

Pyridoxine (Vitamin B6)

If 2 doses of a benzodiazepine do not terminate the seizure activity, a therapeutic dose of pyridoxine should be given serious consideration. Empiric pyridoxine dosing is 5 g intravenously (IV) in an adult and 70 mg/kg IV in a child. This dose may be adjusted, and pyridoxine can be administered on a gram-per-gram basis with isoniazid in cases of known isoniazid ingestion. Pyridoxine administration is specifically intended to ensure that the patient will have adequate quantities of GABA. This situation is critical in hydrazine poisoning and may be effective in other types of poisoning (eg, theophylline). The effect of this therapy should be apparent within minutes of administration. Unfortunately, the infrequent use of this product and the large quantity needed in the management of toxin-related seizures make it unlikely that it will be readily available for administration. Therefore, if seizure activity has not stopped after 10 minutes from onset, it is appropriate to administer a parenteral barbiturate while awaiting pyridoxine. Phenytoin has not been shown to be effective in this setting.[71,72]

Propofol

This unique agent has activity both at the GABA receptor complex and at NMDA receptors. Propofol induces sedation by increasing GABA tone and antagonizing excitatory tone at NMDA receptor.[73] This dual mechanism has a theoretical benefit when treating toxin-related seizures secondary to increased NMDA activity, such as sedative hypnotic withdrawal. Because propofol suppresses neural transmission in a mechanism totally independent of GABA, it can also be instrumental in the treatment of status epilepticus caused by toxins with potent GABA inhibition, such as flumazenil, lindane, and certain pesticides, as well as other toxins, which understandably may not respond to benzodiazepines and barbiturates. Propofol has an extremely quick onset and its effects terminate rapidly. Caution should be used when administering propofol, because it frequently causes respiratory depression. Propofol dosage required for status epilepticus is generally greater than sedation dosing and approaches induction dosing: adults, 2mg/kg-5mg/kg bolus dosing titrating to response. Patients will require endotracheal intubation and ventilation. [74,75]

Barbiturates

The barbiturate with which most clinicians are familiar is phenobarbital. Other barbiturates, such as pentobarbital,[76] have several advantages and should also be considered, particularly in cases of status epilepticus.[77] Pentobarbital dosing is 5–15 mg/kg loading dose over 15 minutes followed by maintenance infusion of 0.5–3 mg/kg/hour. The clear advantages of pentobarbital, thiopental, secobarbital, or other fast-acting barbiturates include greater potency, high lipid solubility, and more rapid onset of peak activity relative to phenobarbital. In addition, pentobarbital's activity at the GABA receptor is less dependent on the presence of adequate normal quantities of GABA, a theoretical benefit in treating seizures induced by toxins that deplete GABA.[78] These fast-acting barbiturates impart a greater risk of respiratory depression and hypotension relative to phenobarbital. Caution is clearly indicated when using any barbiturate after previous treatment with a benzodiazepine. These drugs work synergistically,[79] with benzodiazepines increasing the frequency of GABA chloride channel opening and barbiturates increasing the duration of GABA chloride channel opening.[80] Together, they may cause sedation to the point of respiratory depression or respiratory arrest. If administration of a barbiturate does not successfully terminate the seizure activity, use of propofol at a bolus dose of 1 to 2 mg/kg IV, or an additional dose of barbiturate, should be considered.

Anticonvulsant Infusion and General Anesthesia

If bolus dose administration of barbiturates and propofol is unsuccessful, continuous infusion of an anticonvulsant is recommended. Pentobarbital, midazolam, and diazepam have commonly been used for this purpose. Propylene glycol, used as a diluent for certain parenteral benzodiazepine preparations, is a toxic alcohol that may induce toxicity if given as an infusion. Like other toxic alcohols, such toxicity results in an acidemia.[81,82] Some reports show a benefit to propofol infusion for the treatment of status epilepticus, though further studies are needed.[83,84] Propofol infusion has been anecdotally described as causing a metabolic acidosis, sometimes fatal, by an unknown mechanism.[85] These rare adverse drug events are not a contraindication to use these agents, but do warrant regular laboratory assessment to detect the development of acidosis in patients on such infusions.

General anesthesia with inhaled volatile anesthetics, specifically isoflurane, is considered by some as the last line of therapy for refractory status epilepticus, although there are very few data to support their use.[86,87]

Miscellaneous Anticonvulsants: Phenytoin, Lidocaine, and Chloral Hydrate

Phenytoin has been demonstrated to be ineffective for the treatment of isoniazid-induced seizures and withdrawal seizures. Phenytoin can potentially be harmful when used to treat seizures induced by theophylline or cyclic antidepressants.[46,47,88–90] Alternative anticonvulsants (mentioned earlier) should be considered prior to the administration of phenytoin in patients with undifferentiated toxin-related seizures.

Lidocaine and chloral hydrate have been advocated as third-line therapy for refractory status epilepticus. Lidocaine is a sodium channel blocker similar to phenytoin, and has been demonstrated to increase morbidity and mortality with certain toxins.[91] Chloral hydrate is not available in a parenteral form and is associated with cardiotoxicity.[92] As such, neither of these agents is recommended as therapy for toxin-related seizures.

SUMMARY

Toxin-related seizures are common and have significant associated morbidity and mortality. The appropriate management of toxin-related seizures differs from the management of epileptic seizures in several ways that are presented in **Fig. 2**. The management strategy for toxin-related seizures discussed herein can be safely applied to seizures of unknown etiology or epileptic seizures, but the converse is not true.

KEY CONCEPTS

- The majority of toxin-related seizures respond to benzodiazepine therapy.
- Pyridoxine should be considered in the treatment of status epilepticus of undetermined etiology.
- Phenytoin should not be routinely administered to patients with toxin-related seizures.
- In all patients with seizures, bedside serum glucose determination is critical.
- Drug screens are rarely helpful in the acute management of patients with seizures.

REFERENCES

1. Neundorfer B, Meyer-Wahl L, Meyer JG, et al. [So-called late epilepsy (author's transl.)]. Wien Klin Wochenschr 1978;90(21):765–72 [in German].
2. Granger N, Convers P, Beauchet O, et al. [First epileptic seizure in the elderly: electroclinical and etiological data in 341 patients]. Rev Neurol (Paris) 2002; 158(11):1088–95 [in French].
3. Vespignani H, Legras B, Weber M, et al. [Frequency and semiological evolution of epileptic seizures occurring between 40 and 65 years of age (author's transl.)]. Rev Electroencephalogr Neurophysiol Clin 1981;11(3–4):524–30 [in French].
4. Pesola GR, Avasarala J. Bupropion seizure proportion among new-onset generalized seizures and drug related seizures presenting to an emergency department. J Emerg Med 2002;22(3):235–9.
5. Pascual-Sedano B, Iranzo A, Marti-Fabregas J, et al. Prospective study of new-onset seizures in patients with human immunodeficiency virus infection: etiologic and clinical aspects. Arch Neurol 1999;56(5):609–12.
6. Kunisaki TA, Augenstein WL. Drug- and toxin-induced seizures. Emerg Med Clin North Am 1994;12(4):1027–56.
7. Panganiban LR, Makalinao IR, Corte-Maramba NP. Rhabdomyolysis in isoniazid poisoning. J Toxicol Clin Toxicol 2001;39(2):143–51.
8. Shah BR, Santucci K, Sinert R, et al. Acute isoniazid neurotoxicity in an urban hospital. Pediatrics 1995;95(5):700–4.
9. Belson MG, Kelley TR. Bupropion exposures: clinical manifestations and medical outcome. J Emerg Med 2002;23(3):223–30.
10. Balit CR, Lynch CN, Isbister GK. Bupropion poisoning: a case series. Med J Aust 2003;178(2):61–3.
11. Whyte IM, Dawson AH, Buckley NA. Relative toxicity of venlafaxine and selective serotonin reuptake inhibitors in overdose compared to tricyclic antidepressants. QJM 2003;96(5):369–74.
12. Blumer J, Strong JM, Atkinson AJ Jr. The convulsant potency of lidocaine and its N-dealkylated metabolites. J Pharmacol Exp Ther 1973;186(1):31–6.
13. Spivey WH. Flumazenil and seizures: analysis of 43 cases. Clin Ther 1992;14(2): 292–305.
14. Gueye PN, Hoffman JR, Taboulet P, et al. Empiric use of flumazenil in comatose patients: limited applicability of criteria to define low risk. Ann Emerg Med 1996; 27(6):730–5.
15. van Gelder NM, Sherwin AL. Metabolic parameters of epilepsy: adjuncts to established antiepileptic drug therapy. Neurochem Res 2003;28(2):353–65.
16. Sherwin AL. Neuroactive amino acids in focally epileptic human brain: a review. Neurochem Res 1999;24(11):1387–95.
17. Ben Ari Y. Cell death and synaptic reorganizations produced by seizures. Epilepsia 2001;42(Suppl 3):5–7.
18. Ronne-Engstrom E, Hillered L, Flink R, et al. Intracerebral microdialysis of extracellular amino acids in the human epileptic focus. J Cereb Blood Flow Metab 1992;12(5):873–6.
19. Carlson H, Ronne-Engstrom E, Ungerstedt U, et al. Seizure related elevations of extracellular amino acids in human focal epilepsy. Neurosci Lett 1992;140(1): 30–2.
20. Buckley NA, Dawson AH, Whyte IM, et al. Relative toxicity of benzodiazepines in overdose. BMJ 1995;310(6974):219–21.

21. Ferenci P, Grimm G. Benzodiazepine antagonist in the treatment of human hepatic encephalopathy. Adv Exp Med Biol 1990;272:255–65.
22. Yager JY, Armstrong EA, Miyashita H, et al. Prolonged neonatal seizures exacerbate hypoxic-ischemic brain damage: correlation with cerebral energy metabolism and excitatory amino acid release. Dev Neurosci 2002;24(5):367–81.
23. Kulik A, Trapp S, Ballanyi K. Ischemia but not anoxia evokes vesicular and Ca(2+)-independent glutamate release in the dorsal vagal complex in vitro. J Neurophysiol 2000;83(5):2905–15.
24. Clausen T, Zauner A, Levasseur JE, et al. Induced mitochondrial failure in the feline brain: implications for understanding acute post-traumatic metabolic events. Brain Res 2001;908(1):35–48.
25. Vecsei L, Dibo G, Kiss C. Neurotoxins and neurodegenerative disorders. Neurotoxicology 1998;19(4–5):511–4.
26. Vornov JJ. Toxic NMDA-receptor activation occurs during recovery in a tissue culture model of ischemia. J Neurochem 1995;65(4):1681–91.
27. Chapman AG, Graham JL, Patel S, et al. Anticonvulsant activity of two orally active competitive N-methyl-D-aspartate antagonists, CGP 37849 and CGP 39551, against sound-induced seizures in DBA/2 mice and photically induced myoclonus in Papio papio. Epilepsia 1991;32(4):578–87.
28. Patel S, Chapman AG, Graham JL, et al. Anticonvulsant activity of the NMDA antagonists, D(-)4-(3-phosphonopropyl) piperazine-2-carboxylic acid (D-CPP) and D(-)(E)-4-(3-phosphonoprop-2-enyl) piperazine-2-carboxylic acid (D-CPPene) in a rodent and a primate model of reflex epilepsy. Epilepsy Res 1990;7(1):3–10.
29. Messenheimer JA. Lamotrigine. Epilepsia 1995;36(Suppl 2):S87–94.
30. Rockhold RW. Glutamatergic involvement in psychomotor stimulant action. Prog Drug Res 1998;50:155–92.
31. Peris J, Dunwiddie TV. Inhibitory neuromodulation of release of amino acid neurotransmitters. Alcohol Drug Res 1985;6(4):253–64.
32. Blanchet G, Carpentier P, Lallement G, et al. [Prevention and treatment of status epilepticus induced by soman]. Ann Pharm Fr 1994;52(1):11–24 [in French].
33. Nordt SP, Chew G. Acute lindane poisoning in three children. J Emerg Med 2000;18(1):51–3.
34. Glenn GM, Krober MS, Kelly P, et al. Pyridoxine as therapy in theophylline-induced seizures. Vet Hum Toxicol 1995;37(4):342–5.
35. Tanaka I, Ito Y, Hiraga Y, et al. [Serum concentrations of the pyridoxal and pyridoxal-5′-phosphate in children during sustained-release theophylline therapy]. Arerugi 1996;45(10):1098–105 [in Japanese].
36. Gregus Z, Klaassen C. Mechanisms of toxicity. In: Klaassen C, editor. Casarett and Doull's toxicology: the basic science of poisons. New York: McGraw-Hill Companies; 1996. p. 35–75.
37. During MJ, Spencer DD. Extracellular hippocampal glutamate and spontaneous seizure in the conscious human brain. Lancet 1993;341(8861):1607–10.
38. Berman RF, Fredholm BB, Aden U, et al. Evidence for increased dorsal hippocampal adenosine release and metabolism during pharmacologically induced seizures in rats. Brain Res 2000;872(1–2):44–53.
39. Eldridge FL, Paydarfar D, Scott SC, et al. Role of endogenous adenosine in recurrent generalized seizures. Exp Neurol 1989;103(2):179–85.
40. Kelsey MC, Grossberg GT. Safety and efficacy of caffeine-augmented ECT in elderly depressives: a retrospective study. J Geriatr Psychiatry Neurol 1995;8(3):168–72.

41. Lurie SN, Coffey CE. Caffeine-modified electroconvulsive therapy in depressed patients with medical illness. J Clin Psychiatry 1990;51(4):154–7.
42. Leentjens AF, van den Broek WW, Kusuma A, et al. Facilitation of ECT by intravenous administration of theophylline. Convuls Ther 1996;12(4):232–7.
43. Shannon M, Maher T. Anticonvulsant effects of intracerebroventricular adenocard in theophylline-induced seizures. Ann Emerg Med 1995;26(1):65–8.
44. Huber A, Padrun V, Deglon N, et al. Grafts of adenosine-releasing cells suppress seizures in kindling epilepsy. Proc Natl Acad Sci U S A 2001;98(13): 7611–6.
45. Dunn DW, Parekh HU. Theophylline and status epilepticus in children. Neuropediatrics 1991;22(1):24–6.
46. Goldberg MJ, Spector R, Miller G. Phenobarbital improves survival in theophylline-intoxicated rabbits. J Toxicol Clin Toxicol 1986;24(3):203–11.
47. Blake KV, Massey KL, Hendeles L, et al. Relative efficacy of phenytoin and phenobarbital for the prevention of theophylline-induced seizures in mice. Ann Emerg Med 1988;17(10):1024–8.
48. Taboulet P, Michard F, Muszynski J, et al. Cardiovascular repercussions of seizures during cyclic antidepressant poisoning. J Toxicol Clin Toxicol 1995; 33(3):205–11.
49. Graudins A, Dowsett RP, Liddle C. The toxicity of antidepressant poisoning: is it changing? A comparative study of cyclic and newer serotonin-specific antidepressants. Emerg Med (Fremantle) 2002;14(4):440–6.
50. Jacqz-Aigrain E, Bennasr S, Desplanques L, et al. [Severe poisoning risk linked to intravenous administration of quinine]. Arch Pediatr 1994;1(1):14–9 [in French].
51. Sharma AN, Hexdall AH, Chang EK, et al. Diphenhydramine-induced wide complex dysrhythmia responds to treatment with sodium bicarbonate. Am J Emerg Med 2003;21(3):212–5.
52. Radovanovic D, Meier PJ, Guirguis M, et al. Dose-dependent toxicity of diphenhydramine overdose. Hum Exp Toxicol 2000;19(9):489–95.
53. Spiller HA, Carlisle RD. Status epilepticus after massive carbamazepine overdose. J Toxicol Clin Toxicol 2002;40(1):81–90.
54. Tsai J, Chern TL, Hu SC, et al. The clinical implication of theophylline intoxication in the emergency department. Hum Exp Toxicol 1994;13(10):651–7.
55. Spiegel DA, Dexter F, Warner DS, et al. Central nervous system toxicity of local anesthetic mixtures in the rat. Anesth Analg 1992;75(6):922–8.
56. Olson KR, Kearney TE, Dyer JE, et al. Seizures associated with poisoning and drug overdose. Am J Emerg Med 1993;11(6):565–8.
57. MTBoehnert, Lovejoy FH Jr. Value of the QRS duration versus the serum drug level in predicting seizures and ventricular arrhythmias after an acute overdose of tricyclic antidepressants. N Engl J Med 1985;313(8):474–9.
58. Leutmezer F, Schernthaner C, Lurger S, et al. Electrocardiographic changes at the onset of epileptic seizures. Epilepsia 2003;44(3):348–54.
59. Nelson LS, Hoffman RS. Mexiletine overdose producing status epilepticus without cardiovascular abnormalities. J Toxicol Clin Toxicol 1994;32(6):731–6.
60. Patel MM, Tsutaoka BT, Banerji S, et al. ED utilization of computed tomography in a poisoned population. Am J Emerg Med 2002;20(3):212–7.
61. Earnest MP, Feldman H, Marx JA, et al. Intracranial lesions shown by CT scans in 259 cases of first alcohol-related seizures. Neurology 1988;38(10):1561–5.
62. Zagnoni PG, Albano C. Psychostimulants and epilepsy. Epilepsia 2002;43(Suppl. 2):28–31.

63. Osuide G, Wambebe C, Ngur D. Studies on the pharmacology of d-amphetamine on maximal electroconvulsive seizure in young chicks. Psychopharmacology (Berl) 1983;81(2):119–21.
64. Kleinrok Z, Czuczwar SJ, Kozicka M. Effect of dopaminergic and GABA-ergic drugs given alone or in combination on the anticonvulsant action of phenobarbital and diphenylhydantoin in the electroshock test in mice. Epilepsia 1980;21(5): 519–29.
65. De Sarro GB, De Sarro A. Anticonvulsant properties of non-competitive antagonists of the N-methyl-D-aspartate receptor in genetically epilepsy-prone rats: comparison with CPPene. Neuropharmacology 1993;32(1):52–8.
66. Nevins ME, Arnolde SM. A comparison of the anticonvulsant effects of competitive and non-competitive antagonists of the N-methyl-D-aspartate receptor. Brain Res 1989;503(1):1–4.
67. Munn RI, Farrell K. Failure to recognize status epilepticus in a paralysed patient. Can J Neurol Sci 1993;20(3):234–6.
68. Lowenstein DH, Aminoff MJ, Simon RP. Barbiturate anesthesia in the treatment of status epilepticus: clinical experience with 14 patients. Neurology 1988;38(3): 395–400.
69. I.E.Leppik, Derivan AT, Homan RW, et al. Double-blind study of lorazepam and diazepam in status epilepticus. JAMA 1983;249(11):1452–4.
70. Chamberlain JM, Altieri MA, Futterman C, et al. A prospective, randomized study comparing intramuscular midazolam with intravenous diazepam for the treatment of seizures in children. Pediatr Emerg Care 1997;13(2):92–4.
71. Miller J, Robinson A, Percy AK. Acute isoniazid poisoning in childhood. Am J Dis Child 1980;134(3):290–2.
72. Saad SF, el-Masry AM, Scott PM. Influence of certain anticonvulsants on the concentration of -aminobutyric acid in the cerebral hemispheres of mice. Eur J Pharmacol 1972;17(3):386–92.
73. Orser BA, Bertlik M, Wang LY, et al. Inhibition by propofol (2,6 di-isopropylphenol) of the N-methyl-D-aspartate subtype of glutamate receptor in cultured hippocampal neurones. Br J Pharmacol 1995;116(2):1761–8.
74. Rossetti AO, Milligan TA, Vulliémoz S, et al. A randomized trial for the treatment of refractory status epilepticus. Neurocrit Care 2010. [Epub ahead of print].
75. Rossetti AO, Reichhart MD, Schaller MD, et al. Propofol treatment of refractory status epilepticus: a study of 31 episodes. Epilepsia 2004;45(7):757–63.
76. Van Ness PC. Pentobarbital and EEG burst suppression in treatment of status epilepticus refractory to benzodiazepines and phenytoin. Epilepsia 1990;31(1):61–7.
77. Rashkin MC, Youngs C, Penovich P. Pentobarbital treatment of refractory status epilepticus. Neurology 1987;37(3):500–3.
78. Kaneda M, Wakamori M, Akaike N. GABA-induced chloride current in rat isolated Purkinje cells. Am J Physiol 1989;256(6 Pt 1):C1153–9.
79. Miller LG, Deutsch SI, Greenblatt DJ, et al. Acute barbiturate administration increases benzodiazepine receptor binding in vivo. Psychopharmacology (Berl) 1988;96(3):385–90.
80. Akaike N, Tokutomi N, Ikemoto Y. Augmentation of GABA-induced current in frog sensory neurons by pentobarbital. Am J Physiol 1990;258(3 Pt 1):C452–60.
81. Cawley MJ. Short-term lorazepam infusion and concern for propylene glycol toxicity: case report and review. Pharmacotherapy 2001;21(9):1140–4.
82. Reynolds HN, Teiken P, Regan ME, et al. Hyperlactatemia, increased osmolar gap, and renal dysfunction during continuous lorazepam infusion. Crit Care Med 2000;28(5):1631–4.

83. Brown LA, Levin GM. Role of propofol in refractory status epilepticus. Ann Pharmacother 1998;32(10):1053–9.
84. Prasad A, Worrall BB, Bertram EH, et al. Propofol and midazolam in the treatment of refractory status epilepticus. Epilepsia 2001;42(3):380–6.
85. Kang TM. Propofol infusion syndrome in critically ill patients. Ann Pharmacother 2002;36(9):1453–6.
86. Kofke WA, Young RS, Davis P, et al. Isoflurane for refractory status epilepticus: a clinical series. Anesthesiology 1989;71(5):653–9.
87. Murao K, Shingu K, Tsushima K, et al. The anticonvulsant effects of volatile anesthetics on penicillin-induced status epilepticus in cats. Anesth Analg 2000;90(1): 142–7.
88. Okamoto M, Rosenberg HC, Boisse NR. Evaluation of anticonvulsants in barbiturate withdrawal. J Pharmacol Exp Ther 1977;202(2):479–89.
89. Chance JF. Emergency department treatment of alcohol withdrawal seizures with phenytoin. Ann Emerg Med 1991;20:520–2 [see comments].
90. Callaham M, Schumaker H, Pentel P. Phenytoin prophylaxis of cardiotoxicity in experimental amitriptyline poisoning. J Pharmacol Exp Ther 1988;245(1):216–20.
91. Derlet RW, Albertson TE, Tharratt RS. Lidocaine potentiation of cocaine toxicity. Ann Emerg Med 1991;20(2):135–8.
92. Bowyer K, Glasser SP. Chloral hydrate overdose and cardiac arrhythmias. Chest 1980;77(2):232–5.

Antiepileptic Drugs: The Old and the New

Oliver L. Hung, MD*, Richard D. Shih, MD

KEYWORDS

- Seizure • Benzodiazepine • Overdose • Antiepileptic drugs

During the past decade, 8 new antiepileptic drugs (AEDs) have been approved by the Food and Drug Administration (FDA) for the treatment of seizures (**Table 1**). In contrast, during the preceding 8 decades, only 6 principal AEDs existed for the treatment of generalized and partial seizures, with no new drugs approved from 1978 to 1993. With this new generation of antiepileptic medications, emergency physicians must be familiar with their therapeutic usage and potential adverse reactions. This article provides an overview of these new AEDs as well as the preexisting AEDs.

AEDs: OLD GENERATION
Carbamazepine (Tegretol)

Carbamazepine, which is structurally similar to tricyclic antidepressants, is used to treat partial and generalized tonic-clonic seizures. The mechanism of action of this drug is similar to that of phenytoin, that is, involves slowing the rate of reactivation of voltage-dependent sodium channels after depolarization. The most common side effects are diplopia, headache, dizziness, and nausea. Benign maculopapular or morbilliform rashes occur in 10% of patients.[1] Less common skin eruptions include erythema multiforme and Stevens-Johnson syndrome. A reversible leukopenia also occurs in 10% of patients; however, only 2% of the patients require discontinuation of the medication. Aplastic anemia is rare and occurs in 0.5 per 100,000 treatment-years. Carbamazepine is an inducer of the cytochrome P450 system (3A and 2C9) and increases the metabolism of valproic acid, ethosuximide, corticosteroids, warfarin, phenothiazines, and cyclosporine.

There is no parenteral version of carbamazepine. Oral loading may be possible; one study suggested that a single loading dose of carbamazepine, 8 mg/kg, by suspension or in tablet formulation successfully achieved therapeutic concentrations without significant gastrointestinal (GI) tract side effects within 2 and 5 hours, respectively.[2]

Clonazepam (Klonopin)

The benzodiazepine clonazepam is used in the treatment of absence seizures, myoclonic jerks, and tonic-clonic seizures. However, the tendency of this drug to

Department of Emergency Medicine, Morristown Memorial Hospital, Morristown, NJ, USA
* Corresponding author.
E-mail address: olhung@pol.net

Emerg Med Clin N Am 29 (2011) 141–150
doi:10.1016/j.emc.2010.09.004
0733-8627/11/$ – see front matter © 2011 Elsevier Inc. All rights reserved.

Table 1
Antiepileptic drugs

Drugs	Indications	Serious Adverse Reactions	Drug Interactions
Older Oral AEDs			
Carbamazepine	Partial and generalized seizures	Steven-Johnson syndrome, aplastic anemia	Yes
Clonazepam	Myoclonic seizure	—	No
Ethosuximide	Absence seizure	—	No
Phenobarbital	Partial and generalized seizures	—	Yes
Phenytoin	Partial and generalized seizures	—	Yes
Valproic acid	Absence, partial, and generalized seizures	Toxic hepatitis	No
Newer Oral AEDs			
Felbamate	Partial seizure and Lennox-Gastaut syndrome in children	Aplastic anemia	Yes
Gabapentin	Partial seizure	—	No
Lamotrigine	Partial seizure	Steven-Johnson syndrome	No
Levetiracetam	Partial seizure	—	No
Oxcarbazepine	Partial seizure	—	Yes
Tiagabine	Partial seizure	—	No
Topiramate	Partial seizure	—	No
Zonisamide	Partial seizure	—	No

cause excessive sedation and the eventual development of tolerance to clonazepam has limited its usefulness; it is mainly used for the treatment of refractory myoclonic seizures.

Ethosuximide (Zarontin)

Ethosuximide is considered a first-line AED for patients with generalized absence seizures. The mechanism of action of this drug is related to its ability to reduce calcium currents in specific thalamic neurons. The primary side effects are on the GI tract (nausea, vomiting, abdominal pain) or central nervous system (CNS) (sedation, headache).

Phenobarbital (Phenobarbitone)

Phenobarbital is effective for the treatment of partial and generalized tonic-clonic seizures. Introduced in 1912, phenobarbital is the oldest AED still in use. The primary mechanism of action involves the potentiation of the γ-aminobutyric acid type A (GABA$_A$) receptor. Potentiation is mediated by the promotion of GABA to the receptor and by directly increasing the duration for which the chloride channels remain open. Phenobarbital is the only barbiturate that possesses anticonvulsant properties at sub-hypnotic doses (**Table 2**). Although phenobarbital is as effective as phenytoin and carbamazepine in preventing seizures, it is considered a second-line AED because of its significant CNS side effects, including excessive fatigue in adults and hyperactivity

Table 2
Effects on current medication when treated with newer anticonvulsant

New Anticonvulsants	Carbamazepine	Phenytoin	Valproic Acid
Felbamate	Decrease	Increase	Increase
Gabapentin	None	None	None
Lamotrigine	None	None	None
Topiramate	None	Increase	None/decrease
Zonisamide	None	None	None
Oxcarbazepine	None	None	None
Levetiracetam	None	None/Increase	None
Tiagabine	None	None	None

and aggression in children. Phenobarbital is also a potent inducer of many cytochrome P450 enzymes (1A2, 2A, and 3C), which can result in clinically significant increased metabolism of many medications, including AEDs (carbamazepine, ethosuximide, lamotrigine, tiagabine, zonisamide), antiarrhythmics, antihypertensive agents, corticosteroids, theophylline, estrogens, warfarin, and phenothiazines. Phenobarbital exists in both an oral and a parenteral preparation. However, the administration of loading doses of phenobarbital by intravenous (IV) or oral route is usually impractical and seldom attempted (except in treating patients with status epilepticus) because of the high risk of excessive sedation and respiratory depression.

Phenytoin (Dilantin) and Fosphenytoin (Cerebyx)

Phenytoin is effective for the treatment of partial and tonic-clonic seizures. The drug slows the rate of reactivation of voltage-dependent sodium channels after depolarization. The principal side effects include gingival hyperplasia, hirsutism, acne, and facial coarsening. At plasma concentrations greater than 20 μg/mL, phenytoin may produce neurologic symptoms, including nystagmus, ataxia, dysarthria, and lethargy. Phenytoin is an inducer of the cytochrome P450 system (2C9, 19, and 3A4) and may decrease serum concentrations of benzodiazepines, ethosuximide, felbamate, lamotrigine, oxcarbazepine, tiagabine, topiramate, and zonisamide.

The IV administration of phenytoin may result in hypotension or cardiac arrhythmias (3.5% incidence).[3,4] This risk is related to the rate of administration and the total dose infused and is attributed to phenytoin and its diluents propylene glycol and ethanol. In addition, local irritation from IV phenytoin infusions may result in infusion site reactions (eg, phlebitis, purple glove syndrome, and tissue necrosis). The risk of both hemodynamic complications and infusion site reactions may be decreased by limiting the IV infusion rate to 50 mg/min (25 mg/min in patients with cardiovascular disease) and ensuring that the infusion is given through a well-placed line with a good flow.

Phenytoin has been used as a first-line drug in the management of seizures in the emergency department (ED) because it is formulated in both oral and parenteral preparations and can rapidly achieve therapeutic concentrations. A loading dose of IV phenytoin, 20 mg/kg at 50 mg/min, by continuous infusion can achieve therapeutic concentrations in approximately 30 minutes.[5] Similarly, a therapeutic concentration of phenytoin can be achieved after an oral dose of phenytoin, 20 mg/kg. In an ED study, 64% of patients (N = 44) achieved therapeutic phenytoin concentrations greater than 10 μg/mL within 8 hours after oral loading.[6] Another study evaluated single oral phenytoin administration in both volunteers and hospitalized patients.[7]

All volunteers (N = 19) receiving phenytoin, 15mg/kg, achieved therapeutic phenytoin concentrations of greater than 10 μg/mL within 4 hours. Meanwhile, the hospitalized patients (N = 14) received a higher single dose of oral phenytoin (18.7 mg/kg for males and 24.8 mg/kg for females), and all of them achieved therapeutic phenytoin concentrations within 4 hours and maintained therapeutic concentrations during a 24-hour observation period. The mean peak phenytoin concentrations were 23.9 ± 5.5 μg/mL for males and 21.5 ± 5.1 μg/mL for females.[7]

Fosphenytoin is a parenteral phenytoin prodrug that is metabolized to phenytoin and has the same pharmacologic activity as phenytoin in the treatment of seizures.[8] Fosphenytoin is more water soluble than phenytoin and therefore, does not require dilution with propylene glycol and alcohol. Consequently, this drug lacks phenytoin's serious adverse effects such as hypotension, cardiac arrhythmias, and infusion site reactions. In addition, fosphenytoin can be administered intravenously or as an intramuscular injection. Fosphenytoin is administered in the form of phenytoin sodium equivalents (PSEs). The loading dose is the same as that for phenytoin, 15 to 20 PSEs/kg, but the maximum rate of infusion is much higher, 150 mg/min for adults or 3 mg/kg/min for children. The main advantage of fosphenytoin is the decreased risk of serious adverse effects and its ability to be administered as an intramuscular injection. The main disadvantage of fosphenytoin is its higher cost when compared with phenytoin; however, because fosphenytoin is now available generically, the cost difference is minimal.

Valproic Acid (Depakote)

Valproic acid is unique among the older AEDs because of its effectiveness in treating all types of seizures, including absence, partial, and generalized tonic-clonic seizures. The mechanism of action is similar to that of both phenytoin and carbamazepine in that it prolongs the recovery of voltage-activated sodium channels from inactivation. In addition, valproic acid stimulates GABA synthesis by activating glutamic acid decarboxylase and inhibiting GABA degradation enzymes. The most common side effects are GI tract disturbances, including anorexia, vomiting, tremor, and weight gain. Hepatotoxic reactions include transient reversible elevations of aminotransferases (frequent), reversible hyperammonemia (20% of all patients), toxic hepatitis, and a Reye-like syndrome.[9] The incidence of fatal idiosyncratic hepatotoxicity is 1 in 49,000 adults and 1 in 800 children.[10] Acute pancreatitis has also been associated with the use of valproic acid. In 1997, an IV formulation of valproic acid was approved for use by the FDA. IV valproic acid has been successfully used to treat status epilepticus.[11–13]

AEDs: NEW GENERATION

As a group, the new-generation AEDs seem to be better tolerated, with less-severe side effects (with the exception of felbamate and lamotrigine), and have fewer drug interactions than the traditional AEDs (**Table 3**). Most of these medications are only approved as adjunctive treatments for seizures. Their efficacy as a single treatment of seizures is currently being investigated.

Felbamate (Felbatol)

In 1993, felbamate was approved for the adjunctive treatment of partial seizures in adults and Lennox-Gastaut syndrome in children and adults. This drug is structurally similar to the anxiolytic meprobamate but does not possess any muscle-relaxing properties. The exact mechanism of action of this drug is not known. The drug is

Table 3
Pharmacokinetics of the new AEDs

Drugs	tmax (h)[a]	Half-life (h)	Metabolism	Elimination
Felbamate	1.0–4.0	20.0–23.0	Partly metabolized in liver to inactive metabolites	90% urine (metabolized 40%)
Gabapentin	1.5–4.0	5.0–7.0	None	100% urine
Lamotrigine	2.2–3.0	13.0–30.0	76% glucuronidation	94% urine
Topiramate	2.0–3.0	20.0–30.0	Hydroxylation, hydrolysis, glucuronidation	55%–97% urine, unchanged 62% urine
Zonisamide	2.0–6.0	63.0	Inactive metabolites	—
Levetiracetam	1.0	6.0–8.0	Insignificant, hepatic 24%, enzymatic hydrolysis	91% urine
Oxcarbazepine	4.5	1.0–2.5	10-hydroxycarbazepine (active)	95% urine metabolites
Tiagabine	0.75	7.0–9.0	CYP3A	25% urine (unchanged & metabolites) 63% fecal

[a] Time after dosing when maximum serum concentration is achieved.

postulated to act by interaction with *N*-methyl-D-aspartate class of glutamate receptor.[14] Felbamate inhibits the enzyme CYP2C19 and induces CYP3A4. The concurrent administration of felbamate increases serum concentrations of phenytoin, phenobarbital, and valproic acid and decreases serum concentrations of carbamazepine. The use of felbamate has been associated with the development of aplastic anemia and hepatic failure. The risk of aplastic anemia is estimated at 127 per million users.[15] The risk of hepatic failure is 1 in 30,000 users.[16] Consequently, felbamate has been largely replaced by other alternative AEDs.

Overdose
Few cases of overdose have been reported; overdoses mostly result in a mild CNS depression that resolves with supportive care.[17,18] An overdose of felbamate and valproate has been reported to result in felbamate crystalluria and acute renal failure that was successfully treated with IV hydration.[19] Another overdose of felbamate in a 3-year-old child was associated with restlessness, ataxia, hematuria, and crystalluria.[20]

Gabapentin (Neurontin)
Gabapentin's exact mechanism of action is unknown but is thought to be related to its properties as a GABA agonist and its ability to bind to a specific voltage-sensitive calcium channel in the brain. Gabapentin has been shown to be an effective adjunct for the treatment of partial seizures with or without secondary generalized tonic-clonic seizures.[21] The drug also has been demonstrated to be effective in the treatment of painful neuropathies and is approved for the treatment of postherpetic neuralgia. Investigational uses include monotherapy of refractory partial seizure disorders, treatment of spasticity in multiple sclerosis, and treatment of tremor. Potential psychiatric uses include the treatment of mood disorders and attenuation of disruptive behaviors in patients with dementia.

Gabapentin is not metabolized and is excreted unchanged by the kidneys, making it one of the preferred AEDs in patients with hepatic disease.[21] Adverse reactions are generally mild. Leukopenia has been reported in approximately 1.1% of gabapentin-treated patients.[21] The manufacturer has reported that purpuras frequently occur with gabapentin therapy, which are most often described as bruises resulting from physical trauma.[21] Gabapentin is devoid of any significant drug interactions.[21]

Overdose

Overdose of gabapentin generally results in mild CNS depression. Treatment includes supportive therapy and appropriate GI tract decontamination. Severe withdrawal symptoms have been described in patients after the abrupt cessation of high-dose gabapentin treatment.[22]

Levetiracetam (Keppra)

In 1999, levetiracetam was approved for the treatment of partial seizures with or without secondary generalization. The precise mechanism of action is unknown. Like gabapentin, levetiracetam is not hepatically metabolized and is excreted renally; it is a preferred agent in patients with hepatic disease and should be avoided in patients with renal disease. This drug has no known clinically significant drug interactions and has mild adverse effects.[23] Levetiracetam is available in an IV formulation and is thus a consideration in patients already receiving levetiracetam presenting in status epilepticus secondary to medication noncompliance or in patients with known hepatic disease.

Overdose

Overdose data are limited, but overdose seems to result in mild CNS depression. Treatment of levetiracetam overdose includes supportive therapy, including appropriate GI tract decontamination.

Topiramate (Topamax)

In 1997, topiramate was approved for the treatment of refractory partial seizures in adults. This drug is a derivative of D-fructose, but its mechanism of action is unclear. Topiramate enhances the inhibitory effect of GABA, blocks sodium channels, and antagonizes kainate/AMPA receptor subtype of the glutamate receptor.[24] This drug is also a weak carbonic anhydrase inhibitor. The adverse reactions are generally mild. Patients taking topiramate have a slightly increased risk (1.5%) of developing renal calculi.[24,25] Reports describing the development of acute angle-closure glaucoma in patients on this medication are rare.[24,26,27] Topiramate may reduce the effectiveness of oral contraceptives, increase phenytoin concentrations, and decrease serum digoxin and valproic acid concentrations. Topiramate should be avoided in patients with a history of nephrolithiasis or in those taking carbonic anhydrase inhibitors.

Overdose

Most cases of overdoses of topiramate result in mild CNS toxicity. Two cases involving overdoses of 20 and 40 g of topiramate have resulted in status epilepticus, transient hypotension, metabolic acidosis, and coma. Both patients fully recovered with supportive care.[28] Treatment of topiramate overdose includes supportive therapy, including appropriate GI tract decontamination. IV benzodiazepines should be administered for topiramate-induced seizures.

Tiagabine (Gabitril)

Tiagabine was approved in 1997 for the treatment of partial seizures. It is a chemical derivative of nipecotic acid, a compound found in betel nut. This drug inhibits the reuptake of GABA by binding to recognition sites associated with the GABA uptake carrier. Adverse reactions are generally mild. However, 5% of patients receiving tiagabine experienced some form of status epilepticus and 33% of patients with a history of status epilepticus had a recurrence during tiagabine treatment.[29] Tiagabine is metabolized by the CYP3A4 enzyme but does not seem to affect the serum concentrations of other drugs.

Overdose
Clinical experience with tiagabine overdose is limited. CNS depression and agitation were reported as common symptoms after overdose of up to 800 mg.[29] Status epilepticus after 400 mg ingestion (normal maximum daily dose is 56 mg) has also been reported after tiagabine overdose.[29] A retrospective case series of tiagabine overdoses observed that coma and seizures were common findings. Treatment of tiagabine overdose should include supportive therapy including GI tract decontamination with activated charcoal.[30] IV benzodiazepines should be administered for tiagabine-induced seizures or tiagabine-induced agitation.

Zonisamide (Zonegran)
Zonisamide is a sulfonamide derivative approved in 2000 as an adjunct for the treatment of partial seizures in adults. The exact mechanism of action is not fully understood and is thought to involve the blockade of sodium and T-type calcium channels.[31] Acute psychosis occurred in 2% of patients taking zonisamide.[32] The other side effects include decreased sweating, hyperthermia, and renal calculi. Children seem to be more susceptible to developing hyperthermia than adults. Zonisamide is metabolized by CYP3A4 enzyme and may be affected by other drugs that induce or inhibit this isoenzyme (phenytoin, carbamazepine, and phenytoin). It does not seem to affect the plasma concentrations of other drugs. Few cases of overdose have been reported.

Overdose
Bradycardia, hypotension, respiratory depression, seizures, and coma have been reported after zonisamide overdose.[32] Bradycardia was reported in a 26-year-old woman who became comatose after ingesting an unknown amount of zonisamide, clonazepam, and carbamazepine in a suicide attempt. The zonisamide plasma level was 100.1 μg/mL 31 hours postingestion.[29] Multiple episodes of generalized tonic-clonic seizures as well as cardiac arrest occurred in an 18-year-old woman after a single-drug ingestion of 4.8 g of zonisamide (normal maximum daily dose is 600 mg) in a suicide attempt. The patient's rhythm changed to a perfusing wide complex tachycardia after cardioresuscitative measures but the patient developed severe cerebral edema and brain death.[32]

Lamotrigine (Lamictal)
Lamotrigine was approved in 1998 as an adjunct for the treatment of refractory partial seizures and Lennox-Gastaut syndrome. The exact mechanism of action is not fully understood and may involve the inhibition of glutamate release by inhibition of voltage-sensitive sodium channels.[33] Lamotrigine carries an FDA black box warning for the development of life-threatening rashes. About 10% of patients develop erythema and maculopapular rash. An estimated 1% of pediatric patients and 0.3% of adult patients develop a life-threatening rash (eg, Steven-Johnson syndrome, toxic epidermal necrolysis).[34] The risk is increased with the concomitant administration of valproic acid. The development of any type of bullous or vesicular rash should prompt the immediate discontinuation of this AED. The metabolism of lamotrigine is enhanced by carbamazepine, phenobarbital, and phenytoin and reduced by valproic acid.

Lamotrigine itself does not cause significant induction or inhibition of hepatic drug-metabolizing enzymes.

Overdose

CNS depression is the most common effect of lamotrigine overdose. Overdoses of up to 15 g of lamotrigine have been reported to result in fatalities.[33]

Oxcarbazepine (Trileptal)

Oxcarbazepine was approved in 1999 for monotherapy and adjunct therapy for patients with partial seizures. This drug is the 10-keto derivative of carbamazepine and is quickly metabolized to its active metabolite, 10,11-dihydro-10-hydroxycarba-mazepine. Oxcarbazepine has a mechanism of action similar to carbamazepine and seems less likely than carbamazepine to producing CNS side effects, skin rash, or leukopenia. In addition, monitoring of drug levels and blood cell counts is not necessary. Oxcarbazepine seems to induce hepatic enzymes to a lesser extent than carbamazepine. However, oxcarbazepine seems to be more likely than carbamazepine in causing a dose-related hyponatremia.[35,36]

Overdose

Overdose data are limited. Hypotension, tinnitus, seizures, and bradycardia were reported in one case of oxcarbazepine overdose. A 33-year-old woman developed bradycardia (heart rate = 27/min), tinnitus, hypotension (systolic blood pressure = 60 mm Hg), and a witnessed partial seizure after an unintentional ingestion of oxcarbazepine, 3300 mg, (normal dose is 2400 mg/day) and recovered after supportive therapy.[37]

SUMMARY

With a few exceptions, the new AEDs seem to cause fewer adverse effects and have decreased potential for toxicity in overdose when compared with the older generation of medications. However, their efficacy in preventing seizures has not been fully established. The new drugs are only approved for use for adjunctive therapies for the treatment of seizures. Indications for the ED administration of these drugs are limited, and their administration should only be considered with neurologic consultation.

KEY CONCEPTS

- Fosphenytoin has a better safety profile than phenytoin and can be safely given intramuscularly, with rapid achievement of therapeutic serum levels.

- Valproic acid is available in an IV formulation, which should be used in noncompliant patients on valproic acid who seize, and considered for treating status epilepticus refractory to primary therapies.

- Most AEDs are metabolized in the liver and attention must be given to avoid inducing drug interactions with their use.

- Levetiracetam and gabapentin are renally excreted and can be safely used in patients with hepatic disease.

- In general, the new-generation AEDs do not cause serious morbidity in overdose, and treatment is primarily supportive.

REFERENCES

1. Kramlinger KG, Phillips KA, Post RM. Rash complicating carbamazepine treatment. J Clin Psychopharmacol 1994;14(6):408–13.
2. Cohen H, Howland MA, Luciano DJ, et al. Feasibility and pharmacokinetics of carbamazepine oral loading doses. Am J Health Syst Pharm 1998;55(11):1134–40.
3. Donovan PJ, Cline D. Phenytoin administration by constant intravenous infusion: selective rates of administration. Ann Emerg Med 1991;20(2):139–42.
4. Earnest MP, Marx JA, Drury LR. Complications of intravenous phenytoin for acute treatment of seizures. Recommendations for usage. JAMA 1983;249(6):762–5.
5. Cranford RE, Leppik IE, Patrick B, et al. Intravenous phenytoin in acute treatment of seizures. Neurology 1979;29(11):1474–9.
6. Osborn HH, Zisfein J, Sparano R. Single-dose oral phenytoin loading. Ann Emerg Med 1987;16(4):407–12.
7. Ratanakorn D, Kaojarern S, Phuapradit P, et al. Single oral loading dose of phenytoin: a pharmacokinetics study. J Neurol Sci 1997;147(1):89–92.
8. Fischer JH, Patel TV, Fischer PA. Fosphenytoin: clinical pharmacokinetics and comparative advantages in the acute treatment of seizures. Clin Pharmacokinet 2003;42(1):33–58.
9. Powell-Jackson PR, Tredger JM, Williams R. Hepatotoxicity to sodium valproate: a review. Gut 1984;25(6):673–81.
10. Raskind JY, El Chaar GM. The role of carnitine supplementation during valproic acid therapy. Ann Pharmacother 2000;34(5):630–8.
11. Hovinga CA, Chicella MF, Rose DF, et al. Use of intravenous valproate in three pediatric patients with nonconvulsive or convulsive status epilepticus. Ann Pharmacother 1999;33(5):579–84.
12. Limdi NA, Faught E. The safety of rapid valproic acid infusion. Epilepsia 2000;41(10):1342–5.
13. Sinha S, Naritoku DK. Intravenous valproate is well tolerated in unstable patients with status epilepticus. Neurology 2000;55(5):722–4.
14. Kleckner NW, Glazewski JC, Chen CC, et al. Subtype-selective antagonism of N-methyl-D-aspartate receptors by felbamate: insights into the mechanism of action. J Pharmacol Exp Ther 1999;289(2):886–94.
15. Kaufman DW, Kelly JP, Anderson T, et al. Evaluation of case reports of aplastic anemia among patients treated with felbamate. Epilepsia 1997;38(12):1265–9.
16. Ben-Menachem E. Expanding antiepileptic drug options: clinical efficacy of new therapeutic agents. Epilepsia 1996;37(Suppl 2):S4–7.
17. Hwang TL, Still CN, Jones JE. Reversible downbeat nystagmus and ataxia in felbamate intoxication. Neurology 1995;45(4):846.
18. Nagel TR, Schunk JE. Felbamate overdose: a case report and discussion of a new antiepileptic drug. Pediatr Emerg Care 1995;11(6):369–71.
19. Rengstorff DS, Milstone AP, Seger DL, et al. Felbamate overdose complicated by massive crystalluria and acute renal failure. J Toxicol Clin Toxicol 2000;38(6):667–9.
20. Meier KH, Olson KR, Olson JL. Acute felbamate overdose with crystalluria. Clin Toxicol 2005;43:189–92.
21. Neurontin, gabapentin [package insert]. Neurontin Parke-Davis, New York (NY); 2010.
22. Pittenger C, Desan PH. Gabapentin abuse, and delirium tremens upon gabapentin withdrawal [letter]. J Clin Psychiatry 2007;68(3):483–4.

23. Keppra, levetiracetam [product information]. Keppra UCB Pharma, Smyrna (GA); 2010.
24. Topamax, topiramate [product information]. Janssen Ortho, LLC Guraba, Puerto Rico; 2010.
25. Shorvon SD. Safety of topiramate: adverse events and relationships to dosing. Epilepsia 1996;37(Suppl 2):S18–22.
26. Banta JT, Hoffman K, Budenz DL, et al. Presumed topiramate-induced bilateral acute angle-closure glaucoma. Am J Ophthalmol 2001;132(1):112–4.
27. Rhee DJ, Goldberg MJ, Parrish RK. Bilateral angle-closure glaucoma and ciliary body swelling from topiramate. Arch Ophthalmol 2001;119(11):1721–3.
28. Fakhoury T, Murray L, Seger D, et al. Topiramate overdose: clinical and laboratory features. Epilepsy Behav 2002;3(2):185–9.
29. Gabitril, tiagabine [product information]; 2010.
30. Spiller HA, Winter ML, Ryan M, et al. Retrospective evaluation of tiagabine overdose. Clin Toxicol 2005;43:855–9.
31. Zonegran, zonisamide [product information]. Elan Pharma International Ltd, Eisai Inc, Teaneck (NJ); 2010.
32. Naito H, Itoh N, Matsui N, et al. Monitoring plasma concentrations of zonisamide and clonazepam in an epileptic attempting suicide by an overdose of the drugs. Curr Ther Res 1988;43:463–7.
33. Lamictal, lamotrigine [product information]. GlaxoSmithKline Research Park Triangle (NC); 2010.
34. Guberman AH, Besag FM, Brodie MJ, et al. Lamotrigine-associated rash: risk/benefit considerations in adults and children. Epilepsia 1999;40(7):985–91.
35. Friis ML, Kristensen O, Boas J, et al. Therapeutic experiences with 947 epileptic out-patients in oxcarbazepine treatment. Acta Neurol Scand 1993;87(3):224–7.
36. Pendlebury SC, Moses DK, Eadie MJ. Hyponatraemia during oxcarbazepine therapy. Hum Toxicol 1989;8(5):337–44.
37. Jolliff HA, Fehrenbacher N, Dart RC. Bradycardia, hypotension, and tinnitus after accidental oxcarbazepine overdose [abstract]. Clin Toxicol 2001;39:316–7.

Index

Note: Page numbers of article titles are in **boldface** type.

Emerg Med Clin N Am 29 (2011) 151–158
doi:10.1016/S0733-8627(10)00114-8
0733-8627/11/$ – see front matter © 2011 Elsevier Inc. All rights reserved.

emed.theclinics.com

Moving?

Make sure your subscription moves with you!

To notify us of your new address, find your **Clinics Account Number** (located on your mailing label above your name), and contact customer service at:

Email: journalscustomerservice-usa@elsevier.com

800-654-2452 (subscribers in the U.S. & Canada)
314-447-8871 (subscribers outside of the U.S. & Canada)

Fax number: 314-447-8029

Elsevier Health Sciences Division
Subscription Customer Service
3251 Riverport Lane
Maryland Heights, MO 63043

*To ensure uninterrupted delivery of your subscription, please notify us at least 4 weeks in advance of move.

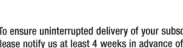
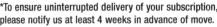

Moving?

Make sure your subscription moves with you!

To notify us of your new address, find your Clinics Account number (located on your mailing label above your name), and contact customer service at:

Email: JournalsCustomerService-usa@elsevier.com

800-654-2452 (subscribers in the U.S. & Canada)
314-447-8871 (subscribers outside of the U.S. & Canada)

Fax number: 314-447-8029

**Elsevier Health Sciences Division
Subscription Customer Service
3251 Riverport Lane
Maryland Heights, MO 63043**

Printed and bound by CPI Group (UK) Ltd, Croydon, CR0 4YY

03/10/2024

01040452-0019